D1187896

2

Essentials of Dermatology

Essentials of Dermatology

J. L. Burton B.Sc., M.D., F.R.C.P.
Reader in Dermatology,
University of Bristol

SECOND EDITION

CHURCHILL LIVINGSTONE
EDINBURGH LONDON MELBOURNE AND NEW YORK 1985

CHURCHILL LIVINGSTONE
Medical Division of Longman Group UK Limited

Distributed in the United States of America by
Churchill Livingstone Inc., 1560 Broadway, New York,
N.Y. 10036, and by associated companies, branches and
representatives throughout the world.

First published 1979
Second edition 1985
    Reprinted 1987

ISBN 0 443 03100 2

British Library Cataloguing in Publication Data

Burton, J.L.
    Essentials of dermatology. — 2nd ed. — (Churchill
    Livingstone medical texts)
    1. Skin — Diseases
    I. Title
    616.5 RL71

Produced by Longman Group (FE) Limited
Printed in Hong Kong.

To Sam Shuster, who showed me that there is more to dermatology than meets the eye.

Preface

This book is based on lectures given to medical students at the
University of Bristol. It is intended to provide, in a readable form,
a firm basis of facts upon which the future general practitioner or general
physician can build by the accumulation of clinical experience.
Forty five colour photographs have been included in this second
edition, and I am extremely grateful to Kirby-Warrick Pharmaceuticals Ltd. (manufacturers of Diprosone, Acnegel and Optimine) who have generously paid the production costs of these
colour plates, thus enabling the book to retain its competitive price.
Forty three new black and white photographs and diagrams have
also been added.

Though these pictures will undoubtedly increase the educational
value of the book, students should be aware that the range of dermatological variants is enormous, and that the 'wallpaper-pattern
matching' method of diagnosis is of limited value. Practical experience, with discussion of the differential diagnosis with an experienced dermatologist, is the best method of acquiring diagnostic competence.

The text has also been updated and expanded (including the
'jokey bits').

Dermatology is a huge subject, and one of its attractions for the
specialist is the fact that rare conditions appear in the clinic relatively frequently, simply because there are so many of them. A
small textbook cannot hope to be comprehensive, and a reference
book may need to be consulted occasionally. The most comprehensive book for clinical dermatology is *Textbook of Dermatology* edited
by A. Rook et al. (4th edition, Blackwell Scientific, Oxford 1985).
For further details of the anatomy and function of normal skin,
Biochemistry and Physiology of the Skin, edited by L. A. Goldsmith
(Oxford University Press, Oxford 1983) is recommended.

1985   J.L.B.

Contents

1

Introduction and principles of diagnosis

There are more than 1000 different skin diseases, most of which may present a variety of appearances. Their nomenclature has, in the past, been confusing and their definition has often been inadequate, since it depended on morphological appearances rather than an understanding of aetiology or pathogenesis. The result has been that many revered physicians have proudly boasted that dermatology is a complete mystery to them. This has been announced in the same tones of smug self-satisfaction which might be used by a poet denying knowledge of the positron, or a plumber grateful for his unfamiliarity with the works of Plato.

Dermatology remains a difficult subject which can properly be learnt only by clinical experience, but nevertheless remarkable progress has been made in the last few decades in our understanding of the pathogenesis and treatment of skin disease, so that dermatology no longer deserves to be treated as a Cinderella science. Dermatology does not occupy an important place in the curriculum of most medical schools, possibly because patients rarely die from skin disease, but there is no doubt of its importance to the general practitioner and his patients. Surveys have shown that practically everyone suffers from at least one skin disease during their life, and 5 to 10 per cent of consultations in general practice are concerned with the skin.

Industrial dermatitis is a major cause of misery in the population, not just because of the symptoms it causes, but also because of loss of work and the consequent financial hardship to the family. Acne vulgaris affects more than half of teenagers, undermining their self-confidence at an age when they feel most insecure. Leg ulcers impair the mobility of many elderly people and place an enormous burden on the country's nursing resources. Psoriasis affects 2 per cent of the population and its effects vary from social embarrassment to lifelong incapacity. These examples merely illustrate the importance of skin disease in the community; they give no indication of the never-ending variety of skin diseases, which is a source of constant fascination for the cognoscenti.

Dermatology is usually regarded as a branch of general medicine, but dermatologists use many surgical procedures (excision, cauterization, freezing, etc.) in their day-to-day work, and their approach to the history and examination differs from that of the general physician. Most skin diseases are confined to the skin, and there is simply not time to perform a full physical examination and system review in every patient. Nevertheless many skin diseases are associated with a systemic abnormality and the art of the dermatologist consists of knowing which patient merits further study. Most dermatologists in a busy practice therefore find it helpful to take a brief history to put the patient at ease and to get a rough idea of the problem. They then examine the skin, and at that stage decide what further history, examination and investigation is necessary. Whereas the neophyte neurologist may take 60 minutes of plodding history and examination to realize that he doesn't know the diagnosis, the trainee dermatologist can arrive at the same conclusion within five minutes! The ability of the experienced dermatologist to diagnose some rare skin disease 'at a glance' because he's seen it before is intellectually frustrating for the student, but clinical expertise of this type becomes increasingly refreshing in these days of laboratory medicine, and dermatology remains one of the few subjects in which the consultant is more likely to be right than his well-read registrar.

Dermatology differs from general medicine too in the patients' marked psychological responses to their diseases. The skin is easily observed and patients often seek attention for what may appear trivial reasons to the objective observer. The skin assumes enormous importance in a person's self-image and its importance as an organ of sexual attraction is well-known. Even a woman built like Raquel Welch will not feel attractive if she thinks she is bald, hairy, spotty, greasy, scaly, wrinkled, red or otherwise dermatologically disadvantaged. Many people believe moreover, with some reasons, that the skin reflects the underlying state of health, and they will often seek reassurance on this point. There is too a widely-held belief, again with some reasons, that the skin is the mirror of the soul, and that many skin diseases are exacerbated by emotional factors. Ever since the days of Job people have looked for a cause for the 'visitation' of their various cutaneous afflictions, and many patients ascribe their disease to something they feel guilty about. The fear of contagion (transmission by touching) is another worry which looms large in the minds of most patients (and medical students), possibly as a relic from the days of the 'unclean' medieval lepers. In fact very few skin diseases other than warts, scabies, fungi, impetigo and syphilis are contagious, and patients should be appropriately reassured on this point. Medical students should observe when the consultant washes his hands and act accordingly.

The net result of these lurking fears and worries is that patients require a great deal of reassurance and explanation. The doctor's task is made more difficult by the fact that the patient can see his skin, and if the treatment is unsuccessful the fact cannot be disguised, although some patients will try their best to join your deception — 'That latest ointment you gave me was marvellous, doctor, it really brought the badness out, and I've got spots now even where I never had them before'.

Principles of dermatological diagnosis

Some skin diseases can be diagnosed immediately, but even in the simplest case the history should not be omitted, for two reasons:
1. It is the patient who seeks treatment, not the rash, and good rapport and understanding will never be achieved without talking to the patient.
2. Appearances can be misleading, and serious mistakes will eventually be made by the dermatologist who ignores the patient's previous medical history and medication.

History

Because of the enormous variety of skin diseases, the history must vary accordingly. Thus it might be reasonable to ask a South American student with red lumps in a line along the forearm if he'd been armadillo-hunting recently (this pastime predisposes to cutaneous sporotrichosis), but this question is not essential for a welder with warts in Wigan. A woman with a bald patch might be asked for details of how she 'permed' her hair, whereas it might be dangerous to ask the welder the same question. On the other hand, if the warts were perianal it would be reasonable to enquire delicately about the possibility of homosexual activity, and even to admire his hairstyle. There is therefore no standard history, but the following 'check-list' may help the inexperienced:
1. When did the trouble start?

2. Where did it start?
3. Has it spread?
4. Does it come and go? If so, do the spots come in crops?
5. Does it itch?
6. Does it ever blister? If so, were the blisters filled with clear fluid?
7. What makes it better?
8. What makes it worse?
9. How does sunlight affect it?
10. What ointments or creams have you used?
11. Do you have any contacts with a similar rash?
12. Any history of previous skin disease?
13. Any history of asthma, or hay fever?
14. Any family history of skin disease, asthma or hay fever?
15. Any previous illnesses?
16. What tablets, medicines or injections have you had in the last six months?

Examination

It has been said that dermatology will have arrived as a science when we have our first blind dermatologist. Until then, it is essential for patients to be examined in a good light, preferably daylight. A torch is essential for use on medical wards, which are often Stygian in several senses. The torch will also be required for examination of the mouth, for if you don't look in it, you'll eventually put your foot in it. A lens is useful as a means of detecting diagnostic minutiae, but it can also be used (like a stethoscope) to give time for a little quiet reflection.

Patients often have a touching faith in the ability of their medical adviser. They will proffer a socially acceptable area of skin such as the dorsum of the hand or the calf and expect him to reach a confident diagnosis from that small area alone. On direct questioning they may deny having any rash elsewhere, even when covered by it. If there is the least doubt about diagnosis or the extent of the disease, patients must be undressed and fully examined, since the diagnosis may depend on the exact distribution of the rash (e.g., nickel allergy affecting the area beneath the metal bra-fastener), or there may be pathognomonic features which present in only one area.

For the beginner it is advisable to examine a dermatosis (skin disease) in the following stages:

1. Describe the *primary lesions* (e.g., macule, papule, vesicle etc.) and any associated *secondary changes* such as excoriation, pigmentation or scarring. Dermatology has its own language, and the following terms may be used to describe these lesions:

Macule: A circumscribed area of discoloration. It may be redder or paler than the surrounding skin, or may be a different colour altogether e.g., blue

Papule: A small raised area. A maculo-papular rash is thus both raised and discoloured

Nodule: A palpable mass larger than 1 cm in diameter

Plaque: A large disc-shaped lesion

Vesicle: A small blister (less than 0.5 cm diameter)

Bulla: A blister more than 0.5 cm diameter

Pustule: A visible accumulation of free pus

Erythema: Redness due to increased skin perfusion

Purpura: Discoloration of the skin or mucosa due to extravasation of red cells. It is distinguished clinically from erythema and telangiectasia by compressing the skin. Purpura does not blanch on pressure

Petechiae: Small purpuric lesions (less than 2 mm diameter)

Ecchymosis: A large extravasation of blood (i.e., a bruise)

Telangiectasia: Permanently dilated, visible small vessels

Weal: An area of dermal oedema. It is usually raised, white, compressible, evanescent and accompanied by a surrounding red 'flare'

Scale: A flake of easily-detached keratin

Crust: An accumulation of dried exudate e.g., serum

Atrophy: A thinning of the skin, often accompanied by loss of normal skin markings and increased translucency

Sclerosis: An induration of the dermis or subcutaneous tissue, often due to increased collagen production

Excoriation: A scratch-mark

Ulcer: A breach in the epidermis, which may range from a small superficial erosion to a massive loss of skin and all the underlying tissues

2. Note the *arrangement* of the primary lesions, relative to each other. They may for example be closely grouped, or diffusely scattered over a wider area, with no clear margin. Sometimes there will be a particular pattern e.g., linear, or annular (ring-shaped) which will narrow the diagnostic field.

3. *Palpate* the lesions gently. This is essential to determine whether they are impalpable, soft, firm or hard, and to elicit ten-

derness and detect heat. It also helps the patient to overcome the 'leper complex' previously mentioned. An added advantage to medical students is that they have to get within arm's-length of the rash, which they otherwise seem reluctant to do. The closer one gets to a rash the more one sees.

4. Having examined the dermatosis in 'close-up', step back and note its overall *distribution* over the whole of the body surface. The skin differs greatly in its anatomy and physiology in various parts of the body, and this helps to localize certain diseases to particular areas e.g., acne vulgaris occurs on the face, chest and back, which are the areas with the largest sebaceous glands. Many other factors (cold, stress, clothing etc.) govern the distribution of a rash however, and some diseases (e.g., pityriasis rosea, p. 124) occur in a particular pattern for reasons which are not currently understood. Hardly any dermatosis occurs 'at random', and the distribution is always of diagnostic importance. It must be remembered however that diseases have not always read the textbooks and may behave in unexpected ways: A rash on the penis is unlikely to be due to 'athlete's foot', but syphilitic chancre of the great toe is not unknown.

5. Note any *special features*. Some diseases have a characteristic hallmark, which suggests the diagnosis. The distinctive feature may be its appearance (e.g., the dimpled pearly papule of molluscum contagiosum), its localization (e.g., sarcoidosis arising in an old scar), its behaviour (e.g., the urtication of a mast cell naevus on rubbing) or some other quality (e.g., favus, a scalp fungus, smells of mice). In a difficult case it may be necessary to search the whole skin surface very carefully for one of these pathognomonic clues.

Further investigations

The investigations, like the history, vary according to the type of case, but they are unlikely to be helpful unless the clinician has narrowed the field to a few diagnostic possibilities.

This is particularly true of the *skin biopsy*, which is difficult to interpret unless full clinical details are given and the pathologist is asked to choose between a limited number of options. In no other subject is it so essential to have good liaison between clinician and pathologist, and many dermatologists either interpret their own slides or have weekly meetings with the histologist to review difficult cases.

The following terms are used to describe some of the histological changes seen in skin disease:

Hyperkeratosis: Thickening of the horny layer

Parakeratosis: Retention of cell nuclei in the horny layer

Acanthosis: Thickening of the epidermis due to an increased number of prickle cells (acanthocytes, but now known as keratinocytes) in the Malpighian layer

Spongiosis: Separation of the keratinocytes by oedema fluid

Acantholysis: Loss of cohesion between keratinocytes due to rupture of the intercellular bridges

Elastotic degeneration: Changes in the dermal collagen which occur in ageing skin in the light-exposed areas. In the late stages whorled masses of disorganized elastin-staining fibres replace the normal collagen

Fibrinoid degeneration: Deposition of eosinophilic material which resembles fibrin. Fibrinoid degeneration in vessel walls is characteristic of necrotizing vasculitis

Necrobiosis: A type of focal necrosis of collagen which leads to the formation of a 'palisading' granuloma

Pigmentary incontinence: The shedding of melanin from the epidermis into the dermis. It is a sign of inflammation or destruction of the epidermal basal layer

In many cases further diagnostic information is obtained by tests of immunofluorescence (p. 200) or special histochemical techniques.

Other investigations used in dermatology include patch tests (p. 180), challenge tests (p. 243), swabs and blister fluid for bacteriology or virology, scrapings for fungus, and examination of brushings from pets (p. 147). Blood tests are relatively unhelpful in dermatological diagnosis unless, as often happens, the disease is secondary to an underlying systemic disease.

2

Disorders of keratinization

PHYSIOLOGY OF KERATINIZATION

The epidermis may be regarded as a biochemical factory for the continual production of keratin. New cells are constantly being produced by mitosis in the basal layer of the epidermis and they become progressively flatter as they ascend through the prickle cell layer (Fig. 2.1).

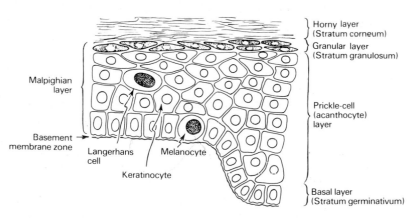

Fig. 2.1 Normal epidermis, showing arrangement of main cell types (diagrammatic)

When they reach the granular layer they undergo a profound metabolic change in which their contents become converted to keratin and they lose their nuclei and die. The flattened squames of dead keratin which are thus formed are then steadily abraded from the skin surface by the physical and chemical trauma of the environment and are shed from the surface as 'dandruff'. The dermis interdigitates with the epidermis in an arrangement reminiscent of a waffle-iron (Fig. 2.2).

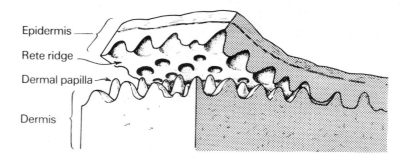

Epidermis —
Rete ridge —
Dermal papilla —➤
Dermis {

Fig. 2.2 Transverse section of a block of skin showing interdigitation of dermal papillae and rete ridges

Cell division in the epidermis is essentially limited to the basal layer. Following each mitosis in the basal layer, one or other of the daughter cells moves into the prickle cell layer and begins to move upwards toward the granular layer. The processes which control this lemming-like migration to differentiation and death are of fundamental importance to the understanding of pathological conditions such as wound healing and psoriasis.

The cell cycle

The study of the kinetics of epidermal proliferation is currently yielding much information about the factors which control cell division and differentiation (Fig. 2.3).

Individual cells have a life cycle which is fairly constant for any specified cell population. It begins at mitosis (M) which is followed by a prolonged period of growth (G_1). After this period the cell has three options:

1. It may leave the cell cycle and undergo metabolic changes leading to differentiation and death, as occurs when the cells reach the granular layer.

2. It may temporarily leave the cell cycle and enter a resting phase (G_0) perhaps analogous to hibernation, during which it neither proliferates nor differentiates, but it can re-enter the cell cycle following suitable stimulation.

3. It may enter a period of active DNA synthesis by the nucleus (S). This is followed by a short resting phase (G_2) prior to mitosis and the start of another cell cycle.

The kinetics of this process can be studied in several ways. H^3-thymidine, which is radioactive, can be injected intradermally and

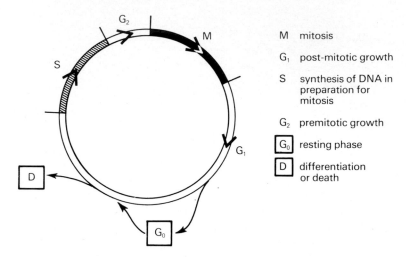

Fig. 2.3 The cell cycle

it is then incorporated into the nucleus of cells in the S phase which can thereafter be identified by autoradiography of a skin biopsy. This technique depends on the fact that the radiation emitted from the tritium (H^3) will cause the silver grains on a photographic plate to become blackened. After some hours the H^3-labelled cells will have entered mitosis and labelled mitoses can also be counted. Another technique depends on the use of a drug such as colchicine which can be used to block cell division at metaphase. It will be appreciated that much data can be accumulated by judicious timing of the injections of H^3-thymidine and/or colchicine, with serial biopsies and counting of cells in various stages of the cell cycle. Appropriate feats of mathematical legerdemain then enable the number of cells in each phase of the cell cycle to be determined. The number of labelled cells in the S phase as a proportion of the total cells is the *labelling index*, and the number of mitotic cells in the cell population is the *mitotic index*. The duration of the complete cell cycle from mitosis to mitosis is known as the *cell turnover time*. This must be distinguished from the *epidermal transit time*, which is the average time taken for a cell to pass from the basal layer through the various epidermal layers until it is shed from the surface of the keratinous layer. The cell turnover time for the epidermal basal cell is about six days, whereas the epidermal transit time is of the order of 28 days. A decrease in the cell turnover time i.e. increased cell proliferation, will thus tend to increase the epidermal thickness, unless there is a corresponding decrease in epidermal transit time.

The control of epidermal proliferation

Repeated rubbing of the skin produces a callosity, and stripping of the superficial layers from the epidermis by the repeated application of adhesive tape (such as Sellotape) produces a burst of mitotic activity in the epidermal basal cell layer. These observations suggest that there must be a local mechanism which controls the rate of cell division in the epidermis. Epidermal proliferation could be due to the release of a mitotic stimulator, but it is more likely that cell division is normally kept in check by an inhibitor of mitosis called a *chalone*. Different tissues produce different chalones and each chalone acts on the tissue which produces it. Chalones are tissue specific but not species specific e.g., epidermal chalone from the pig will inhibit mitosis in the human epidermis but will not inhibit mitosis in the pig liver, whereas human liver chalone will affect pig liver but not human epidermis.

The exact nature of human epidermal chalone is unknown, but there is some evidence to suggest that the 'cyclic AMP cascade' may act as a chalone. Epidermal mitosis is inhibited both by hydrocortisone and by adrenalin and this effect can be explained by their known actions on the cyclic AMP system. This probably accounts for the circadian rhythm in epidermal mitosis, which is inhibited during the day time.

Keratin production

Keratin is an extremely tough, insoluble material which forms the epidermal stratum corneum, hair and nails of humans, and in animals it also forms the horns and hooves. It consists mainly of folded polypeptide chains linked by covalent cross-links. The most important of these links are the disulphide bonds which join two neighbouring cysteine residues of adjacent chains, and it is these bonds which are disrupted and then re-set during the permanent waving process used by hairdressers. The details of the biochemical transition from granular layer cell to horny cell are still obscure, but the process is probably initiated by the release of hydrolytic enzymes from epidermal lysosomes which degrade the cellular organelles. The clumps of keratinized material are eventually shed from the surface of the stratum corneum, probably as a result of the decomposition of the glycosaminoglycans which normally help to cement the living epidermal cells together. If a skin site is protected from all friction by applying a cup to the skin surface for several weeks, a thick mass of moist keratin will accumulate. This may be easily scraped off however, and the underlying stratum corneum is normal, which suggests that the desquamation process occurs at a fixed level in the stratum corneum.

Keratinized epithelium peeled from the skin is pliable as long as it remains moist but it becomes very brittle once it is allowed to dry out. This property of keratin is important in the production of 'chapping' of the skin (p. 186) and surface lipids in the keratin layer help to prevent chapping by decreasing water loss. This explains why regular greasing of the skin is important in the treatment of some types of dry eczema.

PSORIASIS

Psoriasis is a chronic inflamatory skin disease which is characterised by increased basal cell proliferation with a very rapid epidermal cell transit time and this produces plaques of thickened scaly epidermis

The basic cause of psoriasis is unknown, though many biochemical defects have been identified in both the involved and the uninvolved skin, and it is likely that a variety of metabolic and immunological events summate to produce the characteristic psoriatic plaque (see p. 16).

Clinical features

Psoriasis affects 2 per cent of the population. It tends to be familial, it can develop for the first time at any age, and it may relapse or remit spontaneously.

The disease can assume many morphological patterns, and although in many cases it is only a minor cosmetic disability, in severe cases it can cause lifelong misery and incapacity, and occasionally it may even prove fatal.

The characteristic appearance, with multiple, well-demarcated, large, red patches covered by thick silvery-white scales, is easy to recognise. The plaques commonly occur on the knees and elbows but no part of the skin is spared, although mucosal surfaces are rarely involved. Mild itching is common, despite textbook claims to the contrary. The nails are often affected, with distal separation of the nail plates from the nail bed (*onycholysis*), thickening and ridging of the nail plate, and characteristic pits. The following variations occur:

Guttate psoriasis This pattern, with showers of small lesions over the trunk, tends to occur in young people. It is often precipitated by a streptococcal tonsillitis, presumably by an immunological mechanism. The prognosis is relatively good, but if the tonsillitis is recurrent, long-term penicillin may be indicated to prevent relapse of the psoriasis.

Pustular psoriasis This is usually confined to the palms and soles of middle-aged patients. There are localized areas of inflamed skin which are evenly studded with sterile yellowish-white pustules (Fig. 2.4). There may be no psoriasis elsewhere, and the condition is often resistant to treatment, although potent steroid ointments, etretinate, tar preparations, Grenz rays (low-voltage X-rays of poor penetrance) or PUVA therapy (p. 18) may help.

A much rarer form of pustular psoriasis involves the whole body, with malaise, fever and leucocytosis, and this severe form may be fatal. Some authorities believe that generalized pustular psoriasis

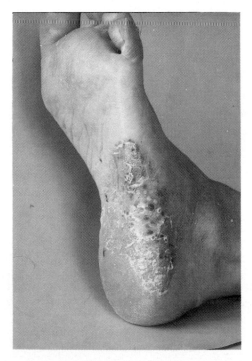

Fig. 2.4 Pustular psoriasis of the palmo-plantar type

may occasionally be precipitated by the use of potent steroid ointments.

Flexural psoriasis Psoriasis localized to the body folds (e.g., beneath the breasts) loses its characteristic scale and may be difficult to distinguish from intertrigo (p. 185) and Candidosis. It tends to occur in the elderly.

Scalp psoriasis Patients complaining of 'severe dandruff' may have psoriasis confined to the scalp. Unlike dandruff (p. 51) scalp psoriasis can be easily felt as thick plaques and it occurs in patches. It may cause bald patches which recover with successful treatment of the psoriasis.

Erythroderma This terms refers to a condition in which more than 90 per cent of the body surface is involved by an inflammatory skin disease such as psoriasis or eczema. Such patients may suffer from a variety of metabolic derangements which are secondary to the skin disease, since they disappear with successful therapy.

Psoriatic arthropathy Arthritis may complicate psoriasis, presumably as an immunological abnormality. Tests for rheumatoid factor are negative, and so this is classed as a sero-negative arthropathy. It is interesting to note that patients with Crohn's disease or ulcerative colitis (both of which can be complicated by sero-negative arthropathy) have an increased risk of developing psoriasis. There are four main clinical patterns of joint involvement.

1. Terminal interphalangeal joints
2. Ankylosing spondylitis and sacro-iliitis
3. Small joint arthritis (e.g., wrists) which mimics rheumatoid arthritis
4. Severe destructive arthritis with marked deformity and osteolysis ('arthritis mutilans').

Mild cases may respond to simple anti-inflammatory drugs but severe cases may need systemic immunosuppressive therapy e.g., methotrexate. Psoriatic arthropathy is more common in patients with psoriatic nail dystrophy.

Napkin psoriasis This starts as a 'nappy rash' which then develops psoriasiform features and may become widespread (Fig. 2.5). It often responds to anti-Candida therapy, and some authorities believe it may be due to Candida or eczema in a baby with a psoriatic predisposition.

Pathology (Fig. 2.6).

The histology of psoriasis shows both acanthosis and hyperkerato-

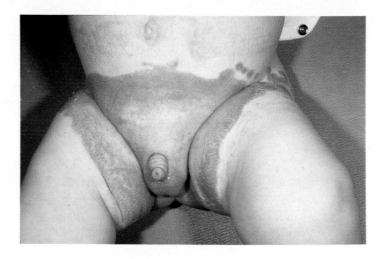

Fig. 2.5 Napkin psoriasis. This baby subsequently developed classical psoriasis

sis. The rete ridges are elongated and thinned with an increased number of mitoses in the basal layer. The blood vessels in the dermal papillae are dilated and there is often a dense leucocytic infil trate in the dermis. Sometimes the neutrophils invade the epidermis to form microabscesses, presumably as a response to a chemotactic stimulus, and this explains why psoriasis sometimes becomes pustular.

The epidermal transit time in psoriasis is decreased to about five days, and so the keratinocytes do not have time to mature properly in the granular layer. As a result, the immature cells in the stratum corneum tend to retain their nuclei (parakeratosis), and stick together to form thick scales.

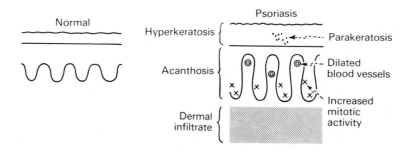

Fig. 2.6 Histology of psoriasis

It has recently been shown that leukotrienes derived from arachidonic acid (Fig. 2.7) are present in the psoriatic epidermis, and these are very powerful chemotaxins for white cells. Abnormalities of prostaglandin metabolism have also been found, and prostaglandins modulate cell division. The rate of epidermal cell division is also dependent on the ratio of the two cyclic nucleotides, CAMP and CGMP, and a decrease in CAMP or an increase in CGMP tends to stimulate mitosis. In psoriatic skin the CAMP:CGMP ratio is decreased and cell proliferation is increased. It may eventually be possible to treat psoriasis with drugs which alter the CAMP:CGMP ratio, or which block lipoxygenase or cyclo-oxygenase enzymes. Benoxaprofen (Opren), recently withdrawn because of toxicity, is one such drug which is effective against psoriasis.

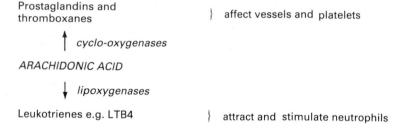

Prostaglandins and
thromboxanes   } affect vessels and platelets

↑ cyclo-oxygenases

ARACHIDONIC ACID

↓ lipoxygenases

Leukotrienes e.g. LTB4   } attract and stimulate neutrophils

Fig. 2.7

Numerous other biochemical defects have been identified in the psoriatic epidermis, including abnormal levels of proteinases, phospholipases, glycogen, etc., but the relationship between these various defects is obscure. Some of the abnormalities are also present in the uninvolved epidermis, and even in the red and white cells of the peripheral blood. This suggests that they are fundamental defects which are not secondary to events in the clinically affected skin.

This is a very active field of research at present, with a constant stream of sophisticated papers adding to our knowledge of the biology of cell division, but despite all this effort, we still do not know the cause of psoriasis.

The familial incidence of psoriasis, and the increased incidence of certain HLA — antigens (e.g., B13) suggest that genetic factors are important. The lymphocytic infiltrate on histology together with the precipitation of guttate psoriasis 10 to 20 days after a streptococcal infection suggest that immunological factors also play a part.

Trauma such as a surgical wound will also trigger psoriasis in the damaged skin, and this has been called the Köbner phenomenon. Sunlight usually helps to clear psoriasis, but a few patients will deteriorate, especially if the skin becomes burnt. Any drug eruption may provoke psoriasis in a predisposed subject, but chloroquine and lithium seem specifically to exacerbate psoriasis, the latter presumably by its known effect on CAMP. Emotional stress tends to exacerbate most inflammatory skin disease, and psoriasis is no exception.

Treatment

The treatment of psoriasis varies with the severity of the disease.

1. *Topical steroids* Most patients with limited psoriasis find that a steroid ointment applied twice daily to the patches will reduce scaling, itching and redness, but the effect is only palliative. The more potent preparations (p. 250) should not be used in infants, or on the face or flexures. For regular use the weakest effective steroid should be used, and many patients find Emulsifying Ointment alone quite useful.

2. *Dithranol* (anthralin) More severe cases will usually respond to treatment with dithranol paste, which acts as a topical cytotoxic drug, and often produces a true remission. The disadvantages of this treatment are that it is tedious to apply, it tends to burn the surrounding normal skin, and it produces a temporary brownish-purple staining of the skin. For best effects, the paste must be stiff, to prevent spread to normal skin, and Lassar's paste forms a good vehicle. The paste must be carefully spread every day over each psoriatic plaque. Starch powder is then sprinkled on the surface of the paste and tubular gauze dressings are applied to keep it in place. In hospital practice the patients usually have a tar bath, every morning, followed by UV irradiation, prior to application of the dithranol (the Ingram regime). The tar bath loosens the psoriatic scales and also enhances the response to the UVR, since tar is a photosensitizer. Patients vary considerably in their response to dithranol, and the concentration may need to be increased during the course of treatment, which usually lasts about 14 days. Suitable concentrations are 0.05 to 0.5 per cent dithranol in Lassar's paste, and patients with pale skin, fair hair and blue eyes, who sunburn easily, will require the lower strengths. Patients must be warned to keep the paste well away from the eyes, since it is irritant, and if the

skin becomes red and inflamed, treatment should be withheld for a day or two, and reinstituted with a lower strength of dithranol.

An alternative method which has recently found favour in some centres is the so-called 'short-contact' dithranol therapy, in which a much higher concentration of dithranol in yellow soft paraffin is applied to the skin for 30 minutes and then washed off. This has the advantage that it can be performed without the necessity for hospital admission, and it avoids the use of dressings during the rest of the day, but it can burn the skin, and should be supervised by a specialist.

Various proprietary preparations of dithranol in a urea-containing base may also be useful in the outpatient management of psoriasis.

3. *Tar and salicylic ointments* Psoriasis of the scalp presents a difficult problem, but various tar shampoos and salicylic acid ointments may help to remove the excessive scale. The following prescription is a useful pomade, to be massaged into the scalp each night:

Salicylic Acid 2%
Solution of coal tar B.P. 6%
Coconut oil 25%
Emulsifying ointment to 100

This preparation, though effective, makes the scalp very greasy, and the hair will need to be shampooed on the following morning.

4. *Systemic cytotoxic drugs* Since psoriasis is characterized by an increased rate of epidermal cell proliferation it is rational to treat it with drugs which inhibit cell division. Drugs such as methotrexate and azathioprine have given good results in suppressing severe psoriasis, but their use is limited by their toxicity for other rapidly proliferating tissues such as the bone marrow. Methotrexate, which has been widely used for patients disabled by psoriasis, has been shown to cause liver fibrosis, but this risk may be diminished by strict abstinence from alcohol and the use of a weekly, instead of a daily, dose of the drug. Careful follow-up is essential, and some experts recommend an annual liver biopsy for patients requiring prolonged methotrexate treatment.

5. *PUVA therapy* This development was stimulated by the observation that psoriasis improves following UV irradiation. The UV wavelengths between the 'sunburn' range (UVB) and visible light normally produce little effect on the skin (p. 156). Certain plant extracts called psoralens are photoactivators, and following ingestion or topical application they will cause the skin to exhibit a sunburn response to the UVA wavelengths, as follows (Fig. 2.8):

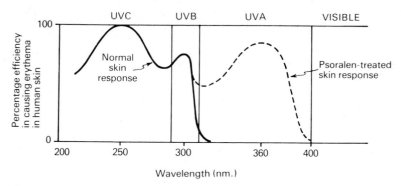

Fig. 2.8 Effect of psoralens on the action spectrum for sunburn

The term PUVA refers to the combination of psoralen therapy with irradiation by lamps which are specially designed to have a very high energy output around 360 nm (i.e., psoralen — UVA). The ingestion of a single dose of methoxypsoralen sensitizes the skin to UVA for about 8 hr. Patients therefore take the tablets at home, and 2 hr later, are irradiated for about 20 min. Some 48 hr later they develop an erythematous reaction which is followed by an attractive golden brown tan. Three treatments each week for several weeks are required to clear the psoriasis, and thereafter maintenance therapy is needed about once a week.

Most centres are at present restricting this treatment to elderly patients or patients with incapacitating psoriasis, since the long-term hazards are uncertain. Psoralens bind to DNA, using the energy of UVA irradiation, and thus inhibit mitosis by preventing DNA replication. Animal experiments suggest that this might considerably enhance the risk of actinic elastosis and skin cancer in later life, but it will be many years before the true risk of this therapy can be accurately assessed. Short-term side-effects include occasional nausea and pruritus and the risk of a servere sunburn reaction. Patients should avoid natural sunlight for 8 hr following psoralen ingestion, and they should wear dark glasses during this time to avoid the theoretical risk of cataract development.

6. *Etretinate* This aromatic retinoid, a vitamin A derivative, has given good results in a variety of disorders of keratinization. It is especially valuable for a rare disease called Darier's disease, and for some rare types of ichthyosis (see below), but it also produces dramatic improvement in some cases of pustular or erythrodermic psoriasis. Its use is limited by its side-effects, since it often causes dryness and cracking of the lips, dryness of the conjunctiva or nasal

mucosa, painful peeling of the palms and soles, and thinning of the hair. It is also teratogenic, and is stored in the body for some months after the treatment is stopped, thus contraception in females should be continued for some months.

The aromatic retinoids, like vitamin A itself, seem to protect against cancer, and since PUVA therapy might cause cancer, the idea of combining a low dose of etretinate with PUVA is attractive. Etretinate has been shown to reduce the dose of irradiation needed to control severe psoriasis, but some experts feel that the side-effects of etretinate outweigh this advantage.

ICHTHYOSIS

Ichthyosis is a common disorder of keratinization in which most of the skin is persistently dry and scaly, and the scales are readily detached. There are several types, with different modes of inheritance.

1. *Ichthyosis vulgaris* (dominant) This type, also called xcroderma, is often mild, with fine flakes of skin which readily desquamate. The knee and elbow flexures are usually spared, and the palmar markings are increased. The condition, which is commonly associated with a tendency to atopic eczema, responds well to the regular application of emollients such as aqueous cream or 50 per cent glycerine in water.

2. *X-linked ichthyosis* (sex-linked recessive) This type, which only affects males, is much less common. The scales are much larger and darker, and the flexures are not spared (Fig. 2.9). Some cases are due to deficiency of a specific enzyme (steroid sulphatase) which affects cholesterol metabolism in the epidermis. These cases respond well to the topical application of cholesterol solution. Pregnant women with this enzyme deficiency fail to metabolize steroid sulphates to oestrogen in the placenta. They therefore have low oestrogen levels and a tendency to a delayed onset of labour.

3. *Ichthyosiform erythroderma* There are several variants of this rare but severe condition which may be associated with spasticity and mental deficiency. The palms are usually hyperkeratotic, and the red scaly skin often has an offensive odour. The response to etretinate therapy may be dramatic.

4. *Acquired ichthyosis* This is a rare type in which ichthyosis occurs for the first time in middle-life. This may be a sign of systemic malignancy, especially lymphoma.

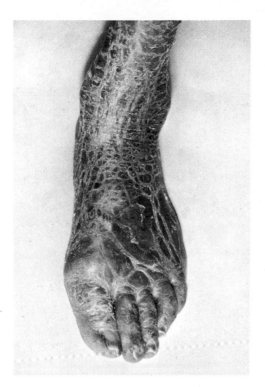

Fig. 2.9 Sex-linked ichthyosis

PALMAR AND PLANTAR KERATOSIS (TYLOSIS)

Several uncommon inherited diseases are characterized by massive lumpy thickening of the palms and soles. In severe cases the condition is both unsightly and disabling. The response to treatment is often disappointing, though 20 per cent salicylic acid ointment will soften the keratin, and oral etretinate is effective in some cases.

DERMATOGLYPHICS

Dermatoglyphics is the study of fingerprint patterns and skin creases. In early fetal life the skin surface is smooth, but as the sweat ducts develop, depressions form in the epidermal surface, and the sweat pores open on the summit of the intervening ridges (Fig. 2.10). These parallel ridges are arranged in two basic types of pattern, namely loops and triradii, which are the bane of the burglar (Fig. 2.11). Their value for identification purposes lies

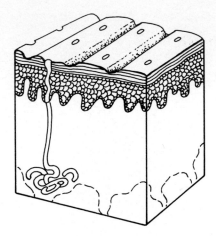

Fig. 2.10 A section of finger-tip skin, showing the opening of the sweat ducts on the ridges

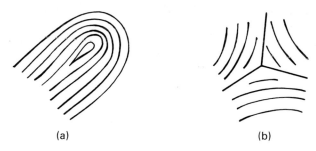

| (a) | (b) |

Fig. 2.11 (a) A loop (b) A triradius

in their precision and their permanence. No two patterns are alike for any two people, and these patterns do not change throughout life; ridge patterns are still visible on some Egyptian mummies.

Any defect of growth in early fetal life is liable to produce changes in the epidermal ridge patterns. These developmental errors can be due to environmental causes (e.g., thalidomide), single gene mutations (e.g., polydactyly), or chromosomal anomalies (e.g., Down's, Turner's and Klinefelter's syndromes).

The dermatoglyphic pattern can therefore provide useful diagnostic clues in a wide variety of congenital diseases. In Down's syndrome (G trisomy), for example, the hands are broad and short and 80 per cent of patients have a distal triradius on the palm, compared with less than 10 per cent of normal subjects (Fig. 2.12). Other

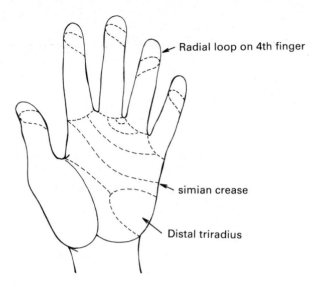

Fig. 2.12 Palmar surface in Down's syndrome

abnormalities may include a transverse 'simian' crease on the palm, one crease (instead of two) on the fifth finger, and a radial facing loop on the fourth finger.

3

Disorders of pigmentation

MELANIN PRODUCTION

Melanin is an inert pigment which is manufactured by the melanocytes in the epidermal basal layer. Its function is to protect cell nuclei from damage by UV irradiation by absorbing energetic particles (free radicals) which would otherwise damage the DNA molecules. On light microscopy it appears brown, but when seen through the intact skin it may look black, and if melanin accumulates in the deeper layers of the dermis it will appear blue, due to the light-scattering effect of the overlying tissue.

Melanin is synthesized from tyrosine in specialised cytoplasmic organelles called melanosomes, which are very numerous in melanocytes (Fig. 3.1).

Tyrosine → dihydroxyphenylalanine → DOPA-quinone → melanin

This reaction is stimulated by tyrosinase enzymes.

The melanosomes, filled with melanin, then pass along the dendritic processes of the melanocyte to be injected directly into the cytoplasm of the neighbouring keratinocytes, where they tend to cluster as a protective cap over the cell nucleus (Fig. 3.1):

Each melanocyte is responsible for producing pigment for its own group of neighbouring keratinocytes. The keratinocytes then migrate upwards through the prickle-cell layer and the melanosomes disintegrate or are eventually shed in the squames from the surface of the horny layer.

Negro skin contains no more melanocytes than Caucasian skin, but the melanosomes produced are larger and are dispersed singly throughout the keratinocytes, instead of being in clumps. The Negro melanosomes are also more resistant to degradation, and intact melanosomes are found in the horny layer.

Melanocyte activity is controlled at a local level by the tyrosinase

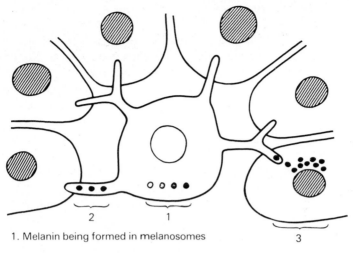

1. Melanin being formed in melanosomes

2. Melanosomes travelling along dendrites

3. Melanosomes being extruded into neighbouring keratinocytes

Fig. 3.1 Pigment production by the melanocyte

enzymes, which are stimulated by UV radiation. Melanin production is also stimulated by various hormones from the pituitary. Melanocyte-stimulating hormone (β-MSH) is part of a larger molecule called lipotrophin. Adrenocorticotrophin (ACTH), which is also derived from the lipotrophin molecule, has a molecular resemblance to β-MSH, and it can also stimulate melanin production. This is of clinical importance in primary adrenal deficiency, in which ACTH secretion is greatly increased.

In the frog, melatonin from the pineal gland makes the skin paler, but the role of melatonin in man is obscure. It may be implicated in the onset of puberty, but it is not known to affect skin colour.

HYPERPIGMENTATION

A. HYPERPIGMENTATION DUE TO MELANIN (hypermelanosis)

Hypermelanosis may be generalized or patchy and the skin may become brown, blue or black.

Generalized hypermelanosis

1. *Genetic* There is considerable variation in skin colour, even in Caucasians, and occasional 'throwbacks' may occur in white families with Negro, Asian or Mediterranean ancestry.

2. *Radiation* Ultraviolet radiation is the best known cause of tanning but other forms of radiation such as X-rays and infra-red rays can also produce pigmentation. A combination of wind and UVR produces a deeper tan than UVR alone, but the mechanism is unknown.

3. *Hormonal* Hypoadrenalism causes diffuse hyperpigmentation as a result of ACTH over-production. A similar change may occur in Cushing's syndrome and may become very marked after adrenalectomy.

Chronic renal failure causes hypermelanosis due to increased circulating β-MSH, since the hormone is normally degraded by the kidney.

Oestrogens also stimulate melanogenesis. Pregnancy causes a generalized increase in skin pigmentation, especially of the nipples and the linea alba, but there may also be a patchy hypermelanosis around the eyes (melasma, chloasma). Oral contraceptives also cause melasma, and in the days of the 'high dose oestrogen' contraceptives, medical students could determine which girls took 'the Pill' by close observation of their facial pigment. Melasma also occurs as an idiopathic condition, and in such cases hydroquinone lotion may be used to depigment the skin.

4. *Metabolic* Any severe wasting disease such as TB or carcinoma can cause diffuse hyperpigmentation.

Malabsorption and biliary cirrhosis are also important causes, and the latter frequently causes severe pruritus in addition.

Haemochromatosis ('bronzed diabetes') sometimes causes a characteristic skin colour, which is due to a combination of melanin and haemosiderin.

5. *Drugs* Arsenic, which was widely used in the past for the treatment of nerve, blood and skin diseases, causes a characteristic diffuse hypermelanosis with multiple small spots of paler normal skin.

Busulphan, used for leukaemia, also causes hypermelanosis, and this drug can also mimic some of the other changes of hypoadrenalism.

Chlorpromazine occasionally causes a slatey-grey discolouration due to a metabolite which binds to melanin.

Patchy hypermelanosis

a. Congenital

1. *Freckles* These appear at about the age of five as small brown macules on light-exposed skin, usually in blonde or red-haired subjects. The melanocytes appear normal on light microscopy, but the melanosomes are abnormally long, and are more active than those in the surrounding skin, and the freckles therefore darken on sun-exposure. Freckled people tend to sunburn easily, and are more likely to develop skin cancer in later life. This so-called 'Celtic complexion' is common in Ireland and Scotland.

2. *Melanocytic naevi* ('moles') (p. 108)

3. *Neurofibromatosis* In this condition there are usually several large macules of a characteristic 'cafe-au-lait' colour, in addition to the soft pedunculated Schwann cell tumours (p. 112). These coffee-coloured patches can be shown on biopsy to contain bizarre giant melanosomes. There may also be freckled pigmentation of the axillae which is virtually pathognomonic for neurofibromatosis.

4. *Peri-orificial lentiginosis* (Peutz-Jegher's disease) This rare autosomal dominant disease is characterized by multiple small deep-brown macules around the mouth, with multiple polyps throughout the intestinal tract. These tend to cause recurrent intussusception and house-surgeons who examine the skin can make the diagnosis preoperatively.

b. Acquired

1. *Lentigines* A lentigo is a brown macule due to a localized increase in epidermal melanocytes. Unlike freckles, lentigines do not darken on exposure to sunlight, but elderly people often develop large lentigines on light-exposed areas.

2. *Post-inflammatory* Any inflammatory skin disease such as eczema or lichen planus may cause hypermelanosis, especially in pigmented races. This is probably due to the release of proteolytic enzymes which activate tyrosinases. The patch of pigment which follows a fixed drug eruption (p. 245) also comes in this category.

Persistent rubbing or scratching can also provoke patchy hypermelanosis.

3. *Acanthosis nigricans* This fascinating condition consists of hyperkeratotic brown areas in the axillae and groins, sometimes with warty lesions elsewhere on the body, and papillomata of the oral mucosa (Fig. 3.2). It almost always indicates underlying malig-

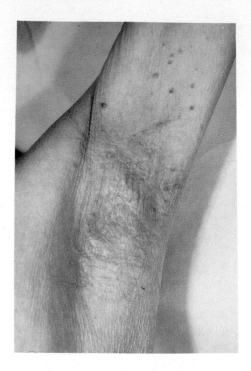

Fig. 3.2 Acanthosis nigricans in a patient with gastric carcinoma

nancy of the gastro-intestinal tract, and tends to regress if the tumour is eradicated. The cause is unknown, but it is presumably yet another endocrine manifestation of malignancy.

Acanthosis nigricans may rarely develop in obesity or acromegaly and even more rarely it may be familial. In these cases it is not a sign of malignancy.

B. HYPERPIGMENTATION NOT DUE TO MELANIN

1. *Jaundice* is a yellow, orange or greenish discoloration due to retention of bile pigments. It is best detected by examination of the sclerae by natural light.

2. *Haemosiderosis* due to iron deposition, causes red-brown discoloration. It may be generalized (e.g., haemochromatosis) or localized in areas of chronic extravasation of red cells (e.g., capillaropathy, venous eczema).

3. *Carotenaemia* causes orange discoloration of keratin and is most marked on the palms. It occurs in a mild form in myxoedema,

and in those (e.g., food faddists) who consume large quantities of carrots.

4. *Ochronosis* is a characteristic blue-black discoloration of cartilage and connective tissue (sclerae, nose and ears). The most important cause is alkaptonuria, a rare defect in amino-acid metabolism which also causes arthritis.

5. *Drugs* e.g., mepacrine (yellow)
          silver (slate-blue)
          gold (blue-grey)
          amiodarone (blue-grey)

6. *Exogenous pigment* may be impregnated in the skin (tattoos, coal dust, grit etc.) or may be merely staining the surface. Many dermatological remedies stain the skin (e.g., dithranol, potassium permanganate, iodine) and general practitioners are occasionally consulted by patients worried by exogenous pigmentation. One of my colleagues was able to reassure a young man that the red ring on his penis was only lipstick.

HYPOPIGMENTATION

Hypomelanosis may be generalized or patchy.

Generalized hypomelanosis. This is relatively uncommon.

1. *Albinism* is due to a congenital inability to form melanin. Patients have fair skin, blonde hair and pink irises. They commonly have poor vision, photophobia and nystagmus, and in tropical countries they run a high risk of developing multiple skin cancers because of their poor protection from UV-induced damage. Several partial forms exist with a variety of metabolic defects such as tyrosinase deficiency.

2. *Phenylketonuria* is due to congenital deficiency of phenylalanine hydroxylase, with consequent accumulation of phenylketones which are toxic to the cerebral neurones. The increased phenylalanine is a competitive inhibitor of tyrosinases, and many patients are therefore attractive blue-eyed blondes who look like angels (Fig. 3.3), but behave like devils because of their mental deficiency and aggression. It is essential to detect this disease at birth, in order to restrict dietary phenylalanine.

3. *Hypopituitarism* causes the skin to become pale because of the ACTH and MSH deficiency. Pallor with axillary hair loss suggests

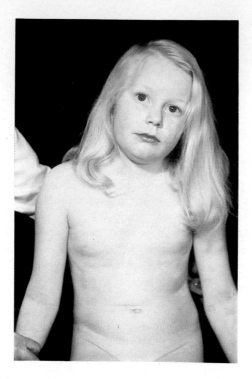

Fig. 3.3 Hypopigmentation due to a block in melanin synthesis in phenylketonuria

the diagnosis. The possibility must be considered in any woman whose periods fail to resume after the birth of a baby.

Patchy hypomelanosis

1. *Vitiligo* This is a common condition in which completely white patches develop due to melanocyte destruction. (Fig. 3.4). It is probably an autoimmune disease. Anti-melanocyte antibodies have been demonstrated, and there is a statistical association with other organ-specific auto-immune diseases such as Hashimoto's thyroiditis, pernicious anaemia and Addison's hypoadrenalism. Vitiligo is also more common in patients with a halo naevus (p. 110), and in alopecia areata, which is also thought to be an auto-immune disease.

Most Caucasian patients in temperate climates require no treatment other than occasional protection of the pale areas from sun-

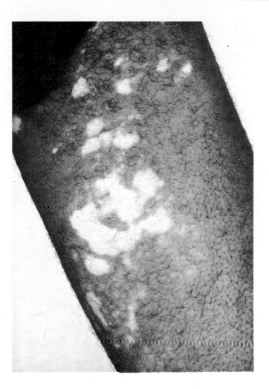

Fig. 3.4 Vitiligo of the thigh

burn. In pigmented races, however, vitiligo is a serious cosmetic problem. In some countries, vitiligo is mistaken by lay people for the depigmented patches of leprosy, and sufferers may become social outcasts, with loss of job and income. In such cases repigmentation can often be induced by oral psoralen therapy followed by regular graded exposure to tropical sunshine. In very extensive cases it may be easier to depigment the remaining areas of normal skin with hydroquinone cream.

2. *Post-inflammatory depigmentation* White patches occasionally follow the resolution of eczema or psoriasis, particularly in pigmented patients. Pityriasis alba is a type of mild eczema often seen in children which characteristically leaves pale patches.

3. *Pityriasis versicolor.* This superficial fungal infection (p. 141) produces multiple, small, slightly scaly, pale macules which become more noticeable after a suntan. The depigmentation is due to a fatty acid (azaleic acid) produced by the fungus, which inhibits tyrosinase activity.

4. *Leprosy*. This disease is not endemic to Britain, but it is seen occasionally in Asian or African immigrants. The tuberculoid form presents as a hypopigmented anaesthetic macule (p. 130).

Other tropical diseases which can cause hypopigmentation include leishmaniasis, yaws, pinta and onchocerciasis.

5. Rarer causes of pale patches include *tuberous sclerosis* (p. 112), *morphoea* (p. 224) and *lichen sclerosus et atrophicus* (p. 193).

4

Disorders of hair and nails

THE HAIR

Structure of hair

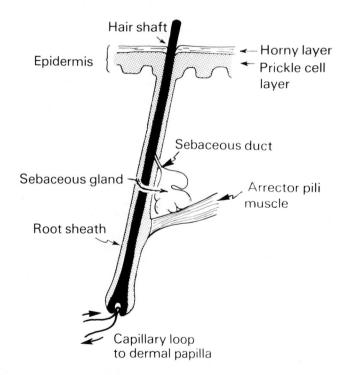

Fig. 4.1 Transverse section of the pilo-sebaceous unit

Each hair follicle consists of an invagination of the epidermis which encloses at its base a small vascular *dermal papilla*. The area of the follicle surrounding the dermal papilla, called the *hair bulb*, is the site of intense mitotic activity which results in the formation of the *hair shaft*.

The hair shaft is composed of inert elongated keratinized cells which are tightly cemented together. This arrangement gives the shaft enormous tensile strength. The keratinous *cortex* which makes up the bulk of the hair shaft is covered by a thin *cuticle*, whose cells overlap slightly, with their free edges pointing upwards. Some hairs (terminal hairs, q.v.) also have a central core called the *medulla* (Fig. 4.2)

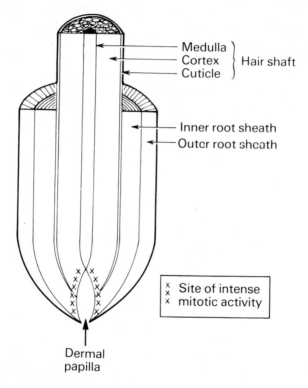

Medulla ⎫
Cortex ⎬ Hair shaft
Cuticle ⎭

Inner root sheath
Outer root sheath

ˣ Site of intense
ˣ mitotic activity

Dermal papilla

Fig. 4.2 Structure of hair

Types of hair

The fetus is covered by a pelt of long soft *lanugo* hair which is shed into the amniotic fluid at about seven months. Lanugo hair is not normally seen after birth except in very premature babies.

Post-natal hair ranges in type from the soft short unmedullated *vellus* hairs (seen to advantage on the thighs of suntanned blondes) to the longer coarse medullated *terminal* hairs of the scalp and eyebrows. Many hairs are of an intermediate type, and it must be remembered that androgens may stimulate a follicle to switch from the production of a vellus hair to a terminal hair. The hairs of the pubic triangle and the axillae are most sensitive to androgen, and the relatively low levels of adrenal androgens produced by the normal female cause these hairs to become terminal at puberty. In the female the upper margin of the pubic hair tends to be horizontal, whereas in the male the hair extends up the abdomen towards the umbilicus. The follicles of the beard and chest area usually require stimulation by higher androgen levels before they produce terminal hair. The distinction between the male and female hair patterns is not absolute however, but is only a matter of degree. Genetic factors are also very important in controlling the hair follicle responses. The end-organ response to a given level of hormonal stimulation may also vary. In the male, body hair tends to increase throughout middle age at a time when the circulating androgen levels may be decreasing. There is also a marked increase in the hairiness of the nostrils and ears in ageing males and the cause of this proliferation is obscure.

Cyclic activity of the hair follicle

Each hair follicle shows intermittent activity i.e., the hair grows to a maximum length, then growth ceases and the hair is shed and replaced (Fig. 4.3).

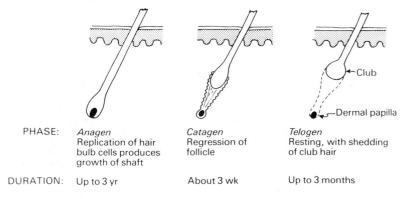

PHASE:	*Anagen* Replication of hair bulb cells produces growth of shaft	*Catagen* Regression of follicle	*Telogen* Resting, with shedding of club hair
DURATION:	Up to 3 yr	About 3 wk	Up to 3 months

Fig. 4.3 The hair cycle

The duration of the active growth phase, *anagen*, varies with the site of the follicle and the age of the subject. Anagen is followed by a short involutional phase, *catagen*, in which the mitotic activity of the hair bulb ceases, and the base of the hair gradually forms an expanded 'club'. This club hair is shed at the end of the inactive *telogen* phase. The next anagen starts when a new hair regrows around the old dermal papilla. Normally less than 1 per cent of hairs are in catagen, but even so, up to 80 hairs may be lost from the normal scalp each day.

In some animals the activity of the hair follicles in synchronized, so that many hairs enter catagen at the same time, and this results in the seasonal 'moulting' of the pelt. In man the follicles act independently of each other, but occasionally a systemic upset such as a pyrexial illness, parturition or severe emotional stress, will stimulate many scalp follicles to enter catagen simultaneously, causing a sudden thinning of the scalp hair two or three months later. The dermatological term for this moulting process, *telogen effluvium* (Fig. 4.4), is likely to increase the alarm of the already distressed patient but she may be reassured that the hair will regrow within a few months.

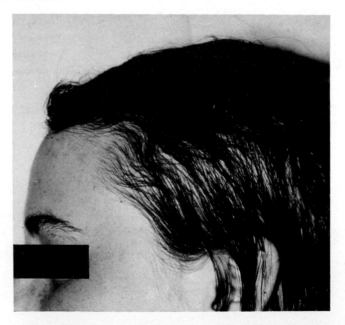

Fig. 4.4 Diffuse alopecia due to telogen effluvium. This developed after severe tonsillitis

Devotees of technological sophistication can measure the rate of hair growth by pulse-labelling with an intra-dermal injection of radioactive cystine-S^{35} which is incorporated into new keratin, but the same answer can be obtained more simply by shaving a small area and measuring the hair length at a later date.

During anagen the cells of the hair bulb have a high mitotic index and cytotoxic drugs therefore affect hair growth. The hair follicles are metabolically very active and they can convert androgens such as testosterone into more active forms such as 5-dihydrotestosterone. This increase in 'tissue androgenicity' is thought to be important in the pathogenesis of male-pattern alopecia and idiopathic hirsutism.

Despite the biochemical complexity of the hair follicle however, patients' complaints about hair can be categorized in the same way that marriage guidance counsellors classify complaints about sex — too much, not enough, or too kinky.

EXCESSIVE HAIR GROWTH

Hirsutism refers to a male pattern of hair growth in the female, e.g., terminal hair in the beard area, with a pubic hairline extending up towards the umbilicus. This androgen-induced pattern should be distinguished from *hypertrichosis* which is the growth of terminal hair in an area which is not normally hairy in either sex, e.g. the forehead.

A. Hirsutism

1. Idiopathic hirsutism

The amount of facial hair in the adult female is subject to considerable racial familial variation, and people therefore differ with regard to what they consider to be abnormal. Hirsutism is very rare among the Japanese and Chinese, whereas women from Wales, Mediterranean countries and India are often hairier than their English counterparts. This 'ethnic' hirsutism presents a difficult problem for doctors called upon to treat immigrants' daughters who have been brought up in a new culture. Idiopathic hirsutism usually begins soon after puberty and patients often have a family history of hirsutism. The condition becomes steadily commoner after the menopause however, and many women eventually grow a moustache if they live long enough.

Idiopathic hirsutism is not a single entity. Some cases may be due to enhanced follicular response to normal circulating androgen levels (probably due to enzymic conversion of testosterone into more active compounds such as dihydrotestosterone). In a normal woman 75 per cent of plasma testosterone originates from the adrenal glands. In hirsutism, a slight increase in plasma testosterone is common, and catheter studies have shown that this comes mainly from the ovaries. Whatever the mechanism, such women are more likely than normal women to suffer from seborrhoea, acne vulgaris, male-pattern alopecia and reduced fertility due to anovulatory cycles.

2. Adrenal disease

The clinical manifestations of hyperplasia or tumour of the adrenal gland depend on the age of onset.

In children with the *congenital adreno-genital syndrome*, the biosynthesis of cortisol is impaired due to an enzyme defect, with consequent overproduction of androgenic steroids. The hirsutism is usually mild and the genitalia may resemble those of the male. This is called female pseudo-hermaphroditism (the true hermaphrodite has gonadal tissue of both sexes, but a pseudo-hermaphrodite has unequivocal gonadal differentiation of one sex, with some of the genital appearances of the other).

In older girls with an *adrenal tumour* there may be a failure of menstruation at puberty and poor breast development. Hirsutism is often marked, and there may besome degree of genital virilization (enlarged clitoris) especially in younger girls. In older women with an adrenal tumour menstruation is irregular, but the hirsutism may be mild.

About a quarter of women with *Cushing's disease* develop hirsutism, and this diagnosis must be considered in any obese hypertensive patient.

3. Ovarian syndromes

The polycystic ovary syndrome (Stein-Leventhal syndrome) consists of the association of hirsutism, obesity, decreased or absent menstrual flow, infertility and polycytic ovaries. These manifestations are very variable however, and the condition probably has a variety of causes. The diagnosis can be confirmed by inspection of the ovaries at laparoscopy. Plasma testosterone levels are often slightly elevated, and the testosterone may originate either from the adrenal or the ovary. Oestrogen production is also increased, and this increases the risk of endometrial problems. There are several types of *virilizing tumour of the ovary*, but fortunately all are rare.

4. Genetic disorders

In *Turner's syndrome* (XO) there may be mild hirsutism, but the short stature, increased carrying angle, webbed neck and broad chest with widely separated nipples will usually suggest the diagnosis.

In *Male pseudo-hermaphroditism* the external genitalia appear female but the ovaries are absent and the vagina is rudimentary.

5. Drugs

A predisposition to hirsutism is produced always by androgens, often by anabolic steroids and occasionally by progestogens and anticonvulsants.

Investigation of hirsutism

The first essential is to exclude any correctable endocrine dysfunction, although most patients will eventually prove to have idiopathic hirsutism.

Authorities differ in the complexity of the investigations they perform to exclude endocrine disease, but a woman with regular periods and a family history of hirsutism is extremely unlikely to have a virilizing tumour. Conversely any young woman whose periods cease, and who develops physical evidence of virilization (enlarged clitoris, hirsutism, seborrhoea and acne vulgaris, male-pattern alopecia, husky voice, etc.) deserves the fullest possible investigation.

Initial investigations in such a virilized patient should include full blood count, plasma testosterone, cortisol and 24 hr urinary steroid excretion (cortisol precursors and derivatives, and adrenal androgens) and skull X-ray (for pituitary size).

Treatment of hirsutism

Treatment is often unsatisfactory unless a correctable endocrine dysfunction is found. Reassurance that no serious disease is present is helpful, but does not remove the patient's complaint.

Most women will have tried proprietary depilatory creams and waxes before visiting the doctor. Depilatory creams cause the hair fibres to swell and produce cleavage of the cystine bridges between adjacent polypeptide bonds as a preliminary to the complete degradation of the hair. Many women find them very irritant.

For 'fuzzy' facial hair, bleaching by dabbing with hydrogen peroxide will make the hair less conspicuous whereas if the hairs are scanty but long the follicles can be destroyed by electrolysis. In this procedure a fine needle is carefully inserted into the individual follicle and a weak electric current is used to destory the root. This method is very time-consuming and a unskilled operator can leave pitted scars. Plucking should be discouraged as it stimulates the follicle to enter the active anagen phase. Waxing is a form of mass plucking.

The simplest way to remove hair is by shaving, but though many women now shave their legs and axillae, they are distressed by the idea of shaving the face. This may be due in some cases to the unspoken fear that they are changing sex, or at least becoming more masculine, and the doctor who browbeats his patient into shaving may amplify this fear. Controlled trials have shown that shaving does not make the hair grow coarser, though most women still believe that it does.

The use of prednisone 5 mg each night, may help to suppress adrenal androgens, and this, in combination with an oestrogenic oral contraceptive may help some patients. The oral antiandrogen drug cyproterone acctate, which was introduced for the treatment of male hypersexuality, has also been successfully used in combination with an oestrogen to treat women with idiopathic hirsutism. It is usually given as the 'reversed sequential' regimen of cyproterone acetate 50 mg daily from day 5 to 15, ethinyl oestradiol 30 μg daily from day 5 to 25 of each menstrual cycle. The contraindications are the same as for any other oral contraceptive, but it should be stressed that pregnancy must be avoided, since a male fetus would probably be feminized, with hypospadias. It usually takes around 6 months before any improvement is seen, and though most patients derive psychological benefit from this treatment, the objective effect on the hirsutism is often less impressive. It is hoped that a topical antiandrogen will eventually be available.

B.Hypertrichosis

Widespread hypertrichosis is a relatively rare condition, but many causes have been documented:

1. Severe infection or malnutrition in children
2. Anorexia nervosa
3. Dermatomyositis (p. 221)
4. Cutaneous forms of porphyria (p. 162)
5. Drugs, e.g., diazoxide, minoxidil
6. Various congenital diseases, e.g. Amsterdam dwarfism
7. Hypertrichosis lanuginosa. This may occur as a rare congenital defect or as a sign of internal malignancy (p. 233)

Localized hypertrichosis may occur as an isolated developmental defect, or in association with pigmented naevi (p. 108). Lumbosacral hypertrichosis ('faun-tail') may be a sign of an underlying vertebral defect.

Inflammatory skin disease, topical steroid therapy and repeated rubbing of the skin may also occasionally stimulate localized hair growth.

ALOPECIA

Long ago, bald foxes and educated dermatologists were common, and so it was decided to designate baldness by a word derived from the Greek for fox — 'alopex'.

1. Male-pattern baldness (Androgenic alopecia)

The common baldness of the ageing male has a characteristic pattern of development. The earliest change is recession of the frontotemporal hairline, followed by thinning on the crown (Fig. 4.5).

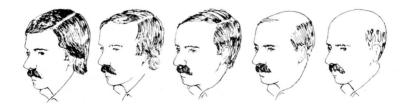

Fig. 4.5 Progression of male-pattern alopecia

Three factors are known to predispose to male-pattern alopecia:

(i) *Increasing age*

Baldness is progressive, and male-pattern alopecia may begin to develop in women after the menopause. Male-pattern alopecia and hirsutism become increasingly common in women over 80, and tonsorial conformity can make it as difficult to distinguish the sexes in geriatric wards as in discotheques.

(ii) *Family history of baldness*

Genetic factors certainly influence both the severity and the age of onset of baldness, but the inheritance is complex and there may be several genotypes.

(iii) *Adequate androgen levels*

A relative deficiency of testosterone protects young women from the development of male-pattern alopecia, even if they inherit the appropriate gene. Males castrated before puberty never become bald but giving testosterone to bald men does not increase the hair loss. The claim that bald men are blessed with enhanced sexual potency may be an old wives' tale, but it must be conceded that old wives are likely to be unusually authoritative in this matter. Although the plasma testoterone levels in bald men are normal, it has recently been claimed that they have a decreased level of the sex-hormone binding globulin compared with their well-thatched contemporaries, so that the amount of non-bound 'active' hormone is effectively increased.

In the balding scalp the terminal hairs are gradually replaced by vellus hairs, and eventually the follicles atrophy to produce the well-known 'billiard-ball' appearance. The pathogenesis of this change is uncertain, but *in vitro* experiments have suggested that bald scalp skin converts testosterone to its more active derivative, 5α-dihydrotestosterone, more readily than similar skin in non-balding men and women. This observation does not explain the paradox that in most situations androgens stimulate vellus hair growth to become terminal, whereas on the scalp the reverse is true.

The treatment of male-pattern alopecia is unsatisfactory. Hair clinics offer a variety of methods for transplanting cash from the anxious patient's wallet to the till, including galvanic stimulation by mini-skirted assistants, rubbing oils, weaving procedures, etc. For pop-stars and others with a Peter Pan personality, punch-grafts transplanted from the hairy occiput to the bald crown will give a better but more expensive result. Topical anti-androgens offer hope for the future, but meantime the virility story is a good one.

For female patients with androgenic alopecia, systemic anti-androgen therapy (cyproterone acetate, see p. 40) should be tried. Though the effects are less obvious to the patient than they are with hirsutism, the rate of loss of hair is often decreased.

2. Chronic diffuse alopecia

In this condition the hair loss is evenly distributed over the whole scalp but with no redness of scaling. It occurs most frequently in adult females. The following causes must be considered but in many cases no cause is found:

1. Telogen effluvium following pyrexia or parturition (p. 36)
2. Severe illness such as malignancy, renal or hepatic failure
3. Hypothyroidism or hypopituitarism
4. Iron deficiency, even in the absence of anaemia
5. Drugs, including antimitotics, antithyroid drugs and all the anti coagulants. Cyclophosphamide has a particularly bad reputation, but remember the oncologist's aphorism 'Better bald coot than dead duck!'

The role of oral contraceptives in causing hair loss is controversial, but there is some evidence that chronic diffuse alopecia occurs more frequently after stopping 'the Pill'. Poisons such as thallium also cause alopecia

6. Mild male-pattern alopecia can be difficult to exclude if there is no recession of the frontal hair line
7. The diffuse form of alopecia areata (pardon the contradictory nomenclature) is easily missed because the usual patchy appearance is not seen, but the presence of exclamation-mark hairs will suggest the diagnosis (see below)

3. Alopecia areata

This is a common disease of unknown aetiology in which sudden hair loss occurs in clear-cut smooth patches of the scalp or beard (Fig. 4.6). The onset may be any age, but it frequently starts in childhood. The bald skin appears normal, but very short broken hair stumps may be visible as black dots or 'exclamation mark' hairs. These are short hairs which when plucked can be seen to have a constriction just above the rounded hair bulb. The appear-

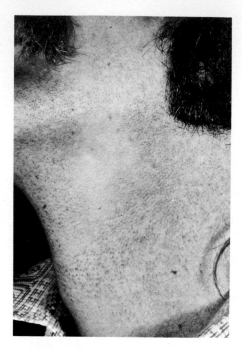

Fig. 4.6 Alopecia areata of the beard area

ance of 'exclamation mark' hairs at the edge of a bald patch is pathognomonic for alopecia areata (Fig. 4.7).

The patches may be single or multiple, and they may enlarge centripetally to become confluent. The hairs are often abnormally loose at the edge of the bald patch during the active stages of the disease. Spontaneous regrowth of hair occurs in the majority of cases, although further attacks may occur in later years. Then new hair growth is often white, but it eventually becomes darker. Occasionally the hair loss extends over the whole of the scalp (*alopecia totalis*) or even the whole body (*alopecia universalis*), including the eyebrows and lashes, and in these cases the prognosis for recovery is poor.

Alopecia areata may be a type of auto-immune disorder since affected hair follicles are surrounded by a heavy lymphocytic infiltrate, the disease remits with steroid therapy, and the patients and their families have a slight increase in the incidence of organ-specific auto-immune diseases (p. 30). Alopecia areata is also occasionally associated with vitiligo and nail pitting, and there is an increased incidence in Down's syndrome.

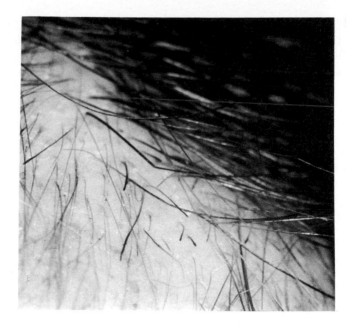

Fig. 4./ Exclamation mark hairs at the edge of a patch of alopecia areata

If spontaneous regrowth has not occurred within a few months and the patches are not too large, triamcinolone injections given intradermally will often stimulate regrowth of tufts of hair in a few weeks. The Panjet apparatus may be used to make the injections painless. Topical application of fluorinated steroids is less effective and even systemic steroids in large doses have only a transient effect. A wig is much safer and more effective, although the loss of eyebrows remains a cosmetic defect.

The repeated application of various irritant and sensitizing chemicals (e.g., dinitrochlorobenzene) to the bald areas induces regrowth of hair in about 30 per cent of chronic cases, but the discomfort and the unreliable results have prevented the widespread introduction of this treatment. It has been suggested that the inflammatory response, with numerous leucocytes being attracted to the area, somehow changes the immunological 'balance', and research is continuing into this intriguing possibility. Topical minoxidil and PUVA therapy have also been claimed to help some patients.

The hair of Marie Antoinette is said to have turned white overnight after hearing her death sentence. For many years scientists declared this trick impossible because pigmented keratin cannot suddenly turn white, but we now know how it is done. Middle-aged people with dark steel-grey hair often have a mixture of black and white hairs. The diffuse form of alopecia areata preferentially affects the black hairs which rapidly fall out, leaving the white hair intact.

4. Scalp infection

(i) *Tinea capitis*, (fungal infection of the scalp), classically produces red scaly bald patches with broken-off hair stumps (Fig. 4.8). The condition usually occurs in children, and the adult scalp is relatively resistant, probably due to the fungistatic effect of fatty acids in sebum. The clinical appearance varies from trivial scaling with a few broken hairs to a huge painful pustular mass called a *kerion*. The severer reactions, which are usually due to a zoophilic fungus (e.g., 'cattle ringworm'), may produce permanent scarring and baldness. The diagnosis of tinea capitis should be confirmed by microscopic and cultural examination of hair since the skin scraping may be negative. The fungal mycelium invades the fully-keratinized hair shaft but cannot invade the hair bulb. When examined under Wood's ultraviolet light the affected hair may show a green fluor-

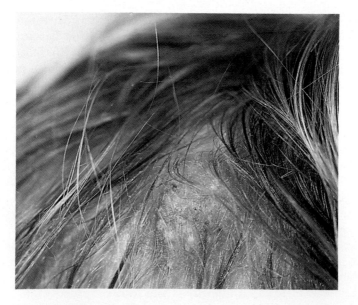

Fig. 4.8 Tinea capitis

escence, and this technique has been used to detect asymptomatic carriers in institutions where tinea capitis has become epidemic. Not all fungi fluoresce and carriers can also be detected by inoculating each subject's hair brush into agar media in a Petri dish. Treatment is with a topical antifungal ointment e.g., tolnaftate and oral griseofulvin (p. 138) and in a severe kerion systemic steroids may also be required to suppress the intense inflammatory response, together with the local application of saline soaks or a starch poultice. Systemic antibiotics may also be needed if secondary bacterial infection has occurred.

(ii) *Bacterial* Pustular folliculitis, furuncles and carbuncles may cause scarring of the scalp which results in a permanently bald patch.

Secondary syphilis produces a variety of skin lesions (p. 132) In the scalp there may be a diffuse alopecia, or small scattered irregular bald spots which lyrical dermatologists describe as the 'glades in the wood' appearance and which the more misanthropic call 'moth-eaten'.

(iii) *Viral* Varicella can produce bald spots around pustules in the scalp but the alopecia is not permanent.

5. Traumatic alopecia

This usually refers to hair loss caused by forcible plucking or the breaking of hair shafts by chemical or physical trauma, but the term may be extended to include scalp damage caused by tomahawks and their latter-day equivalents such as broken bottles, acid burns and spinning machinery.

Excessive scratching or scalp massage can cause broken hair shafts, and babies often develop a patch of occipital alopecia caused by the friction of the pillow before the baby can lift its head (Fig. 4.9). Vigorous repeated brushing with nylon-bristle brushes may also split or weaken the hair.

Various treatments (hot-combs, 'permanent waves', etc.) designed to straighten curly hair or to curl straight hair will do drastic things to the keratin molecule, with consequent fragility of the hair shaft.

Prolonged traction on the hair due to various hairdressing styles, (pony tails, Sikhs, etc.) can produce broken hairs, scaling, erythema and even pustules.

A hair-pulling habit (*trichotillomania*) is not uncommon in nervous children, but it rarely occurs in adults other than mental defectives, madmen and students, who twiddle their hair as they read.

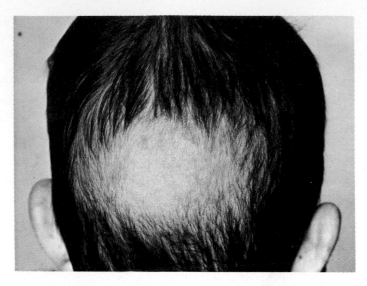

Fig. 4.9 Occipital alopecia in a baby due to rubbing the head on the pillow

6. Other dermatoses

Psoriasis may present with hair loss in the thick scaly plaques in the scalp, but the hair nearly always regrows, following successful treatment of the psoriasis. Severe 'seborrhoeic' dermatitis (p. 184) which can be very difficult to distinguish from psoriasis in the scalp, also causes thinning of the hair.

Lichen planus and discoid lupus erythematosus can both produce scarred areas in the scalp with destruction of the hair follicles (Fig. 4.10). Some dermatologists call this pseudo-pelade.

Many other skin diseases e.g., mycosis fungoides and erythro-derma can involve the scalp to produce a localized or generalized alopecia.

7. Congenital

A whole host of rare congenital diseases cause alopecia, and rainy Monday mornings are occasionally enlivened by their appearance in the outpatient clinic. In some diseases, such as anhidrotic ecto-dermal dysplasia, the defect is widespread and involves internal organs as well as the whole skin, whereas in other cases the defect is confined to the hairshaft. Complex biochemical tests and physical

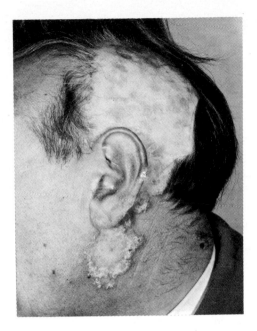

Fig. 4.10 Scarring alopecia due to discoid lupus erythematosus

examination of the hair with the scanning electron microscope may be required to distinguish the various congenital diseases.

Monilethrix is a dominantly inherited condition in which the beaded brittle hair shaft breaks at a length of 1 to 2 cm. In *pili torti* the shaft is flattened and twisted on its own axis, and the reflected light gives the hair a somewhat 'spangled' appearance. *Trichorrhexis nodosa* is a condition in which the hair shaft responds to physical or chemical trauma by forming a nodule which frays and ultimately fractures, leaving a jagged end like a tiny paint brush (Fig. 4.11).

Current work is elucidating the pathogenesis of some of these rare diseases, e.g., *kinky hair disease* (Menke's syndrome), which causes sparse, poorly pigmented hair with retarded mental and physical development, is now known to be associated with abnormal copper metabolism.

The diagnosis of alopecia

The history should refer particularly to the general health, recent illness or stress, the ingestion of drugs or chemicals and a family history of alopecia. The examination should determine:

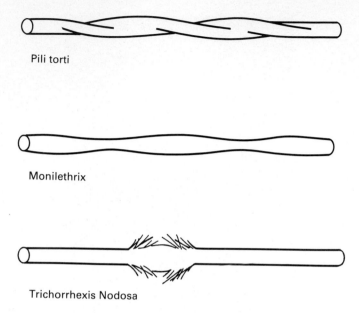

Pili torti

Monilethrix

Trichorrhexis Nodosa

Fig. 4.11 Hair shaft abnormalities seen under a low-power microscope

1. *The pattern of hair loss* This may diffuse, localized (as in male-pattern baldness) or patchy

2. *The state of the scalp* Particular attention should be paid to the presence of erythema and scaling, and the preservation or destruction of hair follicles. The so-called cicatricial alopecias, in which follicles are lost, have a poor prognosis. Minor changes such as atrophy and follicular plugging (p. 218) may help in making the diagnosis

3. *The state of the hair* Hairs should be plucked and examined under the microscope to exclude morphological defects such as pili torti

In addition a full medical examination may be required to detect systemic conditions such as hypothyroidism, secondary syphilis and systemic lupus erythematosus.

Other diagnostic procedures such as examination under Wood's light (UVR), mycological examination of the plucked hairs, and biopsy of the scalp, with serial sectioning and special stains may also be required.

If the patient complains vigorously of hair loss, and yet the hair density appears normal on examination, the possibility of 'dermatological non-disease' (p. 241) must be considered.

Loss of secondary sexual hair (i.e., axillary and pubic hair)

This is common in old age, but in a young woman it may suggest adrenal failure. If this is primary hypoadrenalism the skin will be dark, due to compensatory ACTH production, but if it is secondary to pituitary failure, the skin will be pale.

DISEASES OF THE SCALP

Several conditions other than alopecia can affect the scalp preferentially. The commonest of these is *pityriasis capitis* (dandruff) which consists of the desquamation of small flakes of skin from an otherwise normal scalp. This condition in its mildest form is physiological but in its severer forms the condition shades into 'seborrhoeic' dermatitis (p. 184) with adherent scales and associated erythema and pruritus. Commensal yeasts such as Pityrosporum ovale occur more abundantly in the scalp of patients with dandruff, and this is the probable cause of the condition. Pityriasis capitis responds to a tar shampoo and a steroid-containing scalp application, but treatment may need to be continued indefinitely. Selenium shampoos improve dandruff by reducing the cell turnover rate but they may also increase sebaceous activity. Zinc pyrithione, which is a constituent of many shampoos, is also effective against dandruff, probably by its effect in decimating the yeast population.

Pityriasis amiantacea is a distinctive but uncommon condition in which masses of large silvery scales adhere to the hair and scalp. Psoriasis, seborrhoeic dermatitis and tinea can produce this morphological appearance, but often the condition is idiopathic. It responds well to 5 per cent salicylic acid ointment.

THE NAILS

Each nail consists of a plate of hard keratin which is produced by cell division in the *matrix* at the base of the nail. Part of the matrix is visible through the transparent nail plate as the paler area called the *lunula*. The *cuticle* is an extension of the horny layer of the epidermis on to the nail plate which normally prevents pathogens gaining access to the potential space beneath the *nail fold*.

The finger nails grow much more rapidly than the toe nails. A mark filed on the finger nail at the level of the lunula takes about three months to reach the free margin, whereas for a toe nail the

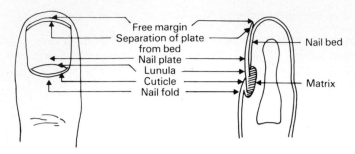

Fig. 4.12 The nail

corresponding time may be up to two years. The nails grow more rapidly in psoriasis, due to the increased cellular proliferation, but the rate of nail growth may be decreased by severe systemic illness. The active nail matrix requires a good blood supply, and digital ischaemia predisposes to nail dystrophy.

A careful inspection of the nails should form part of any medical examination, since the nails can provide a valuable clue to many systemic disorders as well as the patient's emotional state (nail-biters, pickers, etc.), hygiene and even, as Sherlock Holmes pointed out, occupation and social background.

NAIL DYSTROPHIES

The nail may be altered by damage to the matrix, the nail bed or the nail plate itself. Exogenous factors such as infection usually affect only a few nails, whereas endogenous disease is more likely to affect all of the nails, including the toe nails.

1. Onycholysis (Fig. 4.13)

This refers to premature separation of the nail plate from the nail bed. Psoriasis is a common cause, but onycholysis may also be due to trauma, eczema, tinea unguium, photosensitizing drugs, porphyria cutanea tarda or thyroid disease.

2. Koilonychia

This spoon-shaped depression of the nail plate is usually a sign of chronic anaemia, especially in iron-deficiency, but it occasionally follows repeated exposure to strong detergents.

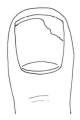

Fig. 4.13 Onycholysis

3. Clubbing (Fig. 4.14)

In the early stages the angle between the nail plate and the posterior nail fold increases to 180° or more, and the matrix is easily depressed and feels spongy. Later the nail curves and the distal phalanx enlarges to produce a 'drumstick' appearance.

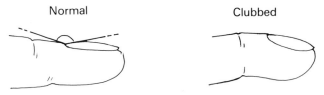

Fig. 4.14 Clubbing

Clubbing is sometimes associated with a painful periostitis of the metacarpals, the distal ulna and radius and this syndrome is called *hypertrophic pulmonary osteoarthropathy*.

The factors involved in the production of clubbing are obscure, but the blood supply to the digits is usually increased.

The following diseases commonly cause clubbing:

Respiratory
1. Bronchial carcinoma
2. Chronic pulmonary suppuration

Cardiovascular
1. Bacterial endocarditis
2. Cyanotic congenital heart disease

Less common causes include:

1. Asbestosis, especially with mesothelioma
2. Fibrosing alveolitis

3. Ulcerative colitis
4. Crohn's disease
5. Cirrhosis
6. Thyrotoxicosis

4. Onychogryphosis

In this condition the nail becomes curved and greatly thickened like a ram's horn. Many causes are due to trauma, and 'ostler's nail', as it was once called, resulted from being stepped on by a horse. Regular chiropody is required, and in severe cases the nail should be surgically removed.

5. Pits

Small depressions in the nail plate are seen commonly in patients with psoriasis. They are due to transient parakeratosis of the nail matrix which thus forms a small area of weak keratin, which is then readily shed. Pits also occur in eczema, lichen planus and alopecia areata.

6. Ridges and grooves

a. *Ridges* may be longitudinal or transverse, and they may be idiopathic or secondary to many dermatoses such as psoriasis, eczema and fungal disease.

b. *Grooves* are usually longitudinal and may be secondary to chemical or mechanical trauma. Picking at the cuticle of the thumb is a common habit which produces a characteristic deformity (Fig. 4.15)

A *mucous cyst* is a collagenous degeneration of the extensor tendon which forms a papule at the base of the bail. It may discharge a

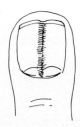

Fig. 4.15 Grooves due to 'picking' at the cuticle

glairy fluid periodically, and pressure from the cyst on the nail matrix often causes a grooved nail plate.

Beau's line is a special instance of a transverse groove caused by a severe systemic illness affecting the matrix. The date of the previous illness can be estimated from the position of the groove in the nail plate (Fig. 4.16) since it takes about 3 to 4 months for the groove to travel from the nail fold to the free margin. In severe cases the nail may be shed.

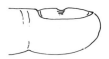

Fig. 4.16 Beau's line

7. Brittle or split nails

This is a common complaint and often no cause can be found, but identifiable causes include repreated wetting of the hands, excessive use of nail varnish remover, iron deficiency, hypothyroidism and digital ischaemia.

8. Shedding of nails

This may follow a severe systemic illness, but is more usually due to a skin disease such as lichen planus or epidermolysis bullosa. The forthright promulgation of unacceptable political views in totalitarian states is also a predisposing factor.

9. Discoloured nails

The colour of the nail may be altered by changes in the matrix, nail bed, nail plate or by external applications (usually in epidemics resulting from the whims of fashion).

(i) *A blue-black nail* is commonly due to a subungual haematoma.

Paronychia associated with Pseudomonas causes a blue-green discoloration, and cytotoxic drugs occasionally produce transverse black bands in the nail.

Patients with a pigmented skin often have a longitudinal streak in the nails. In Caucasians this is much less common, and it should raise the possibility of a subungual malignant melanoma. A longitudinal nail biopsy is sometimes advisable to exclude this condition.

(ii) *Brown nails* are usually due to exogenous staining by cigarette smoke, or to applications such as potassium permanganate solution.

A *subungual exostosis* often causes a reddish-brown appearance of the nail plate in an area which is tender on pressure. Many cases are mistaken for fungus disease, but an X-ray of the phalanx is diagnostic.

Small brown linear streaks in the nail plate may be due to 'splinter' haemorrhages. They occur classically in bacterial endocarditis, but they can be caused by trauma in healthy manual workers.

(iii) *Yellow nails* are often seen in dermatoses such as psoriasis and tinea unguium which produce thickened abnormal keratin.

The yellow nail syndrome is a rare disease in which the nails are small, curved, shiny, yellow and slow-growing, due to defective lymphatic drainage. The defect also involves the lungs, and may predispose to pulmonary infections and pleural effusions.

(iv) *White nails* are clinically a sign of hypoalbuminaemia, especially in cirrhosis but they occur in many other general medical illnesses. In chronic renal failure the white area may be confined to the proximal half of the nail plate (the 'half and half' nail). Hypoalbuminaemia, renal failure and other metabolic disturbances (e.g., cytotoxic drugs) may also produce transverse white bands parallel to the lunula.

Small *white spots* in the nail plate are common. They are said to be due to air pockets in the keratin. They are not a sign of calcium deficiency, and they do not respond to the liberal ingestion of jellies of any flavour.

DISEASES OF THE NAIL FOLD

1. Chronic paronychia

In this condition loss of the cuticle leads to colonization of the space beneath the nail fold by Candida or bacterial pathogens. The nail fold becomes red, tender and swollen, and gentle pressure often causes a bead of pus to exude from beneath the fold. The nail plate often becomes discoloured brown or bluish-black. Predisposing causes include digital ischaemia and frequent immersion of the hands in water. Paronychia is an occupational hazard of bakers, cleaners and bar-tenders.

Treatment

It is essential to keep the hands as dry as possible. Suitable local applications include nystatin ointment and 2 per cent thymol in chloroform but resolution is slow and relapses are common.

2. Ingrowing toe nails

In this condition, which is often due to tight shoes, a spicule of nail grows into the lateral nail fold, causing the production of granulation tissue, with subsequent pain and sepsis.

Treatment

Mild cases can be managed conservatively by cauterizing the granulation tissue with silver nitrate, soaking the feet to soften the nail, and carefully trimming the offending spicule, but severe cases may need radical surgery to prevent recurrence.

3. Herpetic whitlow (p. 118)

4. Periungual erythema

This can be a valuable pointer to a collagen-vascular disease such as lupus erythematosus, dermatomyositis or systemic sclerosis. The dilated and tortuous capillaries can be readily seen with a hand lens, or even more easily with an ophthalmoscope set at +40, and a drop of immersion oil on the nail fold.

5

Disorders of the pilo-sebaceous unit

SEBACEOUS GLAND ANATOMY AND PHYSIOLOGY

Hair follicles and sebaceous glands cover the entire skin surface apart from the palms and soles, the lips and the genital mucosae. Each sebaceous gland drains into a hair follicle via the sebaceous duct and together they constitute the '*pilo-sebaceous unit*'. Sebaceous glands are particularly large and active on the head and neck and the back and front of the chest.

Sebum is produced by a *holocrine* process, i.e., the cells at the periphery of the gland break down and are completely converted into lipid secretion as they move to the gland centre, whence they are excreted through the sebaceous duct, and into the hair follicle. This contrasts with the process of *eccrine* secretion, in which the cells remain intact (e.g., eccrine sweat glands) and *apocrine* secretion in which only a portion of the cell cytoplasm is shed (e.g., apocrine sweat glands). The rate of sebum production thus depends on the size of the glands and their rate of cellular proliferation, and this is regulated by hormonal stimulation. Androgens, particularly dihydrotestosterone, are the most potent stimulants of sebum production, and sebaceous glands only become active at puberty. Other hormones such as thyroid hormone and growth hormone also stimulate sebum production, and this explains why grease production tends to be maximal in male acromegalics and minimal in females with hypothyroidism. Oestrogens decrease sebum production, but this inhibitory effect is overcome by relatively small amounts of testosterone, so that *seborrhoea* (excessive sebum production) can occur in otherwise normal women. Another condition which can cause seborrhoea is Parkinsonism, and in this case the grease production can be decreased by L-dopa therapy. The mechanism is unknown, but one intriguing possibility is that a pituitary sebotrophic hormone is produced in excess in Parkinsonism, and this can then be switched off, via the hypothalamus, by L-dopa. This 'hypophysis hypothesis' awaits confirmation.

Sebum probably serves little useful purpose in man, as shown by the fact that children produce virtually no sebum, yet have healthy and attractive skin and hair. Sebum has a mild fungistatic effect which explains why children are more susceptible than adults to tinea infection (p. 136). In some animals sebum contains vitamin D precursors which can be reabsorbed as vitamin D following UV irradiation, but this appears not to be the case in man. It has also been suggested that seborrhoea might be of evolutionary advantage because it might indirectly boost the development of immune competence. Sebum provides an ideal breeding-ground for the so-called 'acne bacillus' (*Propionibacterium acnes*, or *Corynebacterium parvum*) which immunologists use as an immunity-boosting organism. Malignant melanoma is less common in acne sufferers, and this might be because their immune responses are better able to deal with the incipient melanoma and to eradicate it.

ACNE VULGARIS

This chronic inflammatory disease of the pilo-sebaceous unit is characterized by the development of comedones (blackheads), erythematous papules and pustules on the face, chest and back. There may also be deep cystic lesions (Fig. 5.1), often tender, which eventually resolve to leave pitted scars.

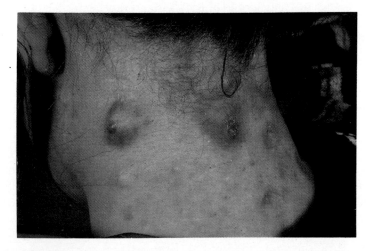

Fig. 5.1 Acne cysts

Incidence

Acne is so common during adolescence that it is abnormal not to be a sufferer. More than half of British teenagers develop acne severe enough to warrant therapy, and for minor grades of acne, with only a few comedones and an occasional pimple, the prevalence exceeds 90 per cent. 'Pimples, shimples, so long as the boy's got puberty,' as Granny used to say.

Pathogenesis

Older texts suggest that acne is due to a combination of deficiencies (e.g., exercise and defaecation) and excesses (e.g., chips and masturbation). The pathogenesis is indeed complex, but these are no longer thought to be the crucial factors.

The initial event is the activation of the sebaceous glands by androgenic stimulation at puberty. Most acne patients have a greasy skin, and there is a good statistical correlation between the sebum excretion rate and the severity of acne. Acne moreover is confined to the skin areas which bear large sebaceous glands. *Seborrhoea* is not the only cause however, for not all subjects with seborrhoea get acne and the sebum excretion rate remains fairly constant throughout life, whereas acne prevalence declines rapidly after adolescence. Colonization of the pilo-sebaceous unit by the anaerobic *Propionibacterium acnes* is also important in the pathogenesis of acne. This bacillus, which uses sebum as a substrate, is present in enormous numbers in the follicles of subjects with a greasy skin. The organism produces lipases which break down the triglycerides in sebum to form *free fatty acids*. These in turn are known to be comedogenic i.e. they will produce blackheads when applied to the epidermis of the rabbit ear. *Comedones* are produced by a defect in the keratinization of the follicular epidermis, so that the squames or keratin, instead of being shed and carried to the surface in the sebum stream, adhere to each other to form a cheesy mélange of keratin, bacteria and sebum which completely or partially blocks the follicle (Fig. 5.2)

Acne may thus be considered to be due to *cohesive hyperkeratinization* of the lower part of the hair follicle. Cytoplasmic organelles called *membrane coating granules* which appear to contain hydrolytic enzymes are necessary for the normal desquamation of keratin, and these granules are known to be sparse in comedones experimentally induced by the application of free fatty acids.

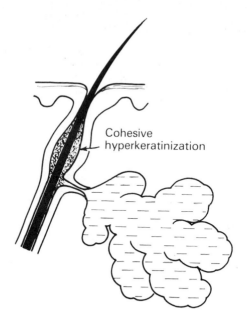

Fig. 5.2 Early stage in comedo formation

Once formed, the comedones lurk in the skin for months or even years, until they are expressed, or until some factor (as yet unknown) initiates the inflammatory response which produces the acne papule. An early event in the inflammatory process is the formation of a breach in the follicular epithelium, around which neutrophils accumulate, and recent work has shown that the comedo contents are both chemotactic and cytotoxic (Fig. 5.3). Immune responses may be invoked, with complement fixation, and in the later stages the reaction may become granulomatous.

Clinical types

1. Adolescent acne

This often begins when the sebaceous glands first become active, and the development of small comedones on the chin at the age of 8 or 9 years is one of the first harbingers of puberty. The severity peaks at around 14 to 18 years and thereafter the disease gradually subsides, though a few unfortunates continue to be plagued into middle age. Though acne is so common as to be normal, the combination of severe acne with hirsutism in a female should suggest

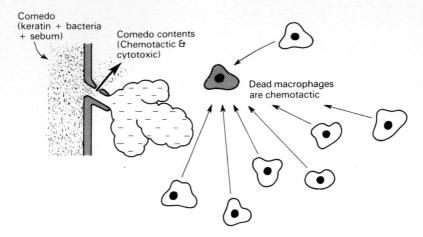

Fig. 5.3 Inflammation in acne vulgaris

the possibility of virilization (p. 38). About 30 to 50 per cent of females with severe acne have increased androgen production; though in males with severe acne the levels of androgen are normal.

Acne vulgaris tends to wax and wane and various precipitating factors have been incriminated. There is often a *'pre-menstrual flare'* each month in females, which may be due to water retention causing follicular obstruction. Nervous stress (e.g., quarrels and exams) may provoke a crop of inflamed lesions, and many patients also blame particular foods such as chocolate or cheese, though scientific proof of this is lacking. Sunlight usually helps the condition, though a few patients find the reverse.

'Acne conglobata' is a devastating form of acne usually seen in men around the age of 20. The back becomes covered in huge suppurating crops of cysts which eventually heal leaving large pink 'tissue-paper' scars. A few patients with acne conglobata have been found to have XYY chromosomes.

'Keloid acne' is another variant of acne vulgaris in which the scars become hypertrophic and keloidal (p. 80).

2. Infantile acne

Many babies develop a few small comedones, but rarely the infant may develop severe acne is which persists for several months or years. It is important to examine the genitalia to exclude precocious puberty and to avoid giving tetracyclines, since these will stain the teeth.

A *comedo naevus* is a rare developmental defect which causes a well demarcated patch of blackheads to develop during childhood.

3. 'Acne excoriée des jeunes filles'

This delightful label is applied to minimal acne in an adolescent girl which provokes an inordinate desire to scratch and 'pick' at the lesions. It is said to be the result of deep-seated psycho-sexual tension which can be unearthed by appropriate probing. Such interviews are invariably interesting but rarely therapeutic.

4. Occupational acne

Various complex *halogenated hydrocarbons* such as chlor-naphthalene can cause a severe and persistent type of acne called *chloracne*. These chemicals occur in various industries (e.g., as electrical insulators) and they may be accidentally produced and disseminated by chemical explosions such as the Seveso disaster in Italy, which liberated dioxin. Other causes of occupational acne include *tar*, which provokes the production of comedones and *mineral oils* which cause comedones and a superficial folliculitis, especially by contact with oil-soaked overalls. Acne developing in an unusual distribution in a middle-aged person should always suggest the possibility of an occupational cause. Comedones are not uncommon in elderly men however, particularly around the eyes in association with solar elastosis induced by chronic exposure to UVR (p. 79). Other forms of radiation e.g., radiotherapy are also comedogenic.

5. Drug-induced acne

(i) *Glucocorticoids and ACTH* sometimes provoke a widespread papular eruption on the trunk which mimics acne vulgaris, though comedones, cysts and scars rarely occur.

(ii) *Anticonvulsants* often seem to make acne worse, but some authors claim that epilepsy itself can be associated with seborrhoea and acne.

(iii) *Iodides (in cough mixtures) and bromides (sedatives)* can cause a very florid pustular drug rash, though this is not true acne vulgaris.

6.   Cosmetic-induced acne

Moisturizing creams and cheap pomades can cause comedones at the anointed site (Fig. 5.4). Some of the preparations contain free fatty acids, which are comedogenic.

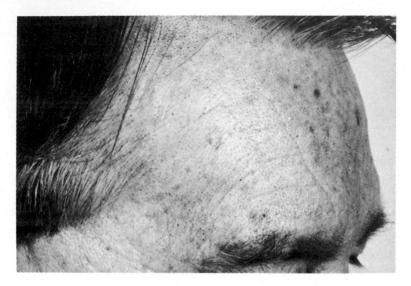

Fig. 5.4 Comedones due to repeated application of a greasy pomade

7.   Acne induced by occlusion

Maceration and friction of the skin caused by 'hippie' head-bands, rucksack straps etc. often produces a band-like localization of acne lesions. Soldiers posted to a tropical climate often develop a very severe exacerbation of their acne, and this 'tropical acne' may be partly due to occlusion of the follicles by surface maceration. Sticking-plaster occlusion can be used to provoke folliculitis experimentally, and this is associated with proliferation of the cutaneous bacteria.

Treatment of acne

Some doctors regard acne as trivial, and dismiss patients with the breezy reassurance that 'You'll soon grow out of it'. In fact it is a major cause of misery in the teenage population, and the psychological distress it induces is often out of all proportion to the visible cosmetic disability. Acne occurs at an age when patients are emotionally most vulnerable, and full explanation and active therapy are essential to prevent scarring of the psyche as well as the skin.

Topical therapy

1. *Benzoyl peroxide* is effective. It has a peeling effect which may help to unblock the follicles, and it also reduces the bacterial population of the skin.

2. *Retinoic acid* is a vitamin A derivative which helps to remove comedones by producing a burst of mitotic activity in the base of the follicle. The comedones are thus pushed out from below, but this treatment often causes irritation and a transient exacerbation of the inflammatory lesions.

3. *Antibiotics* (e.g., topical chloramphenicol or clindamycin) and *antiseptics* may help, presumably by their effect on Propionibacteria.

Systemic therapy

1. Oral oxytetracycline 250mg bd before meals on a long term basis is the treatment of choice for moderate or severe acne. The drug, which accumulates preferentially in the pilo-sebaceous units, is bacteriostatic and it decreases free fatty acid concentrations in the sebum, and also inhibits neutrophil chemotaxis. In resistant cases, the dose may be increased, but this enhances the risk of gastro-intestinal side-effects, especially diarrhoea due to Candida overgrowth of the bowel. Other side-effects are rare, even when the drug is used for several years.

2. Tetracycline does not help all patients, and alternatives which may be tried include *trimethoprim* (*1 Tab.b.d.*) and *erythromycin*. Clindamycin is also effective but carries the risk of inducing a severe colitis.

3. The new vitamin A derivative, *13-cis retinoic acid* (isotretinoin), is extremely effective for severe cystic acne. A course of 3 or 4 months treatment will cause a prolonged reduction in sebum production and a corresponding improvement in the acne. Side-effects include dryness and cracking of the lips, which can be helped by the application of Vaseline (petrolatum), and a tendency for the blood lipids to be increased. The drug is also teratogenic, and in female patients contraception must be ensured.

4. *Oral contraceptives* which are predominantly oestrogenic will reduce sebum excretion, and they are particularly helpful for the

pre-menstrual 'flare' of acne. Progestogenic preparations however tend to make acne worse.

In female patients with severe acne, antiandrogen therapy (see p. 40) may also be considered. There is also a new combined preparation (Diane) which contains a large dose of oestrogen, 50 μg, but only 2 mg of cyproterone acetate. This reduces the rate of sebum secretion by around 30 per cent and is beneficial for mild or moderate acne.

5. Dapsone which interferes with the 'complement cascade' (p. 170) sometimes decreases the inflammatory response in acne.

Other measures

Dietary restriction is not worthwhile unless the patient notices an improvement when particular foods (e.g., dairy products) are avoided. Some physicians seem to burden their patients with impossible diets so that the inevitable transgressions will allow them to provide a self-righteous explanation for the recalcitrance of the disease.

Ultra-violet radiation is helpful, provided a dose which produces slight peeling is used.

Triamcinolone acetonide injected intra-dermally is useful for speeding the resolution of acne cysts. *Freezing* with liquid nitrogen may also be helpful.

Dermabrasion is a type of 'surgical sandpapering' which is useful for a few carefully selected, quiescent cases with deep pitted scars, but it does not help the majority of acne patients, and it carries the risk of causing hyperpigmentation.

ROSACEA

This common chronic disease of unknown aetiology is characterized by diffuse facial erythema with inflamed papules and pustules. The red skin appears tense and shiny, and close inspection will often reveal telangiectasia. Despite claims to the contrary, seborrhoea is not a feature of rosacea, but the skin may look greasy because it is shiny (Fig. 5.5). This appearance is due to lymphoedema, which is occasionally very marked, with considerable swelling of the forehead and peri-orbital areas. Rosacea is usually confined to the face, though it may spread on to the bald scalp and rarely even on to the upper arms.

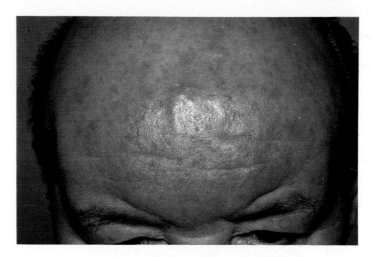

Fig. 5.5 Rosacea, showing the characteristic shiny erythema studded with papules

The condition mainly affects middle-aged and elderly subjects, and it may be distinguished from acne vulgaris by the absence of comedones and scars. It is often exacerbated by exposure to sunshine or heat, and the patients sometimes complain of facial flushing which may be precipitated by emotion, alcohol or hot food.

About one third of patients with rosacea suffer from inflammation of the eyes. Conjunctivitis is the commonest lesion, but blepharitis, scleritis and even keratitis may occur. The latter is painful and can cause corneal ulceration and blindness. Occasionally the ocular manifestations precede the development of the rash.

Rhinophyma is a characteristic florid hypertrophy of the lower third of the nose, with marked erythema, telangiectasia and dilated follicular orifices (Fig. 5.6). The sebaceous glands are markedly increased in size, due to a decrease in the turnover time of the cells which form the lipid. It is often, but not always, accompanied by rosacea, and despite the popular appellation of 'grog-blossom nose' it is not the result of alcoholic over-indulgence.

Pathogenesis of rosacea

The histology of the red skin shows oedema and dilated blood vessels in the upper dermis, with a tendency to solar elastosis (p. 79). Biopsy of the papules shows a dense inflammatory infiltrate of lymphocytes and histiocytes with occasional giant cells and a tendency

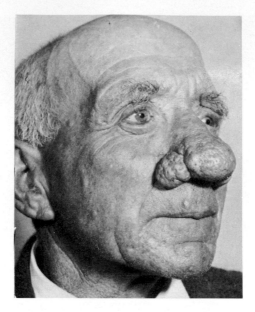

Fig. 5.6 Rhinophyma

to granuloma formation. The histology may resemble tuberculosis but no acid-fast bacilli are found and the disease does not respond to anti-tuberculous drugs. Opinions differ as to whether the hair follicles are preferentially involved in the inflammation. Some experts consider that rosacea is not a disease of the pilo-sebaceous unit, even though the sebaceous glands are considerably enlarged in rhinophyma.

The aetiology of rosacea is unknown and many hypotheses, ranging from something nice in the diet to something nasty in the woodshed, have been proposed and discarded. Demodex folliculorum is a mite which may be found in rosacea and in normal skin, but the evidence that it causes rosacea is far from convincing. A likelier story is that repeated vascular dilation or damage by UV or infra-red radiation releases inflammatory and chemotactic chemicals which trigger off an inflammatory explosion. Television violence has not yet been incriminated.

Treatment

Oral oxytetracycine 250 mg bd for several months reduces the papules and pustules but is relatively ineffective against the erythema.

It presumably acts by its known effect in decreasing leucocyte chemotaxis. Alternative antibiotics which may be helpful include metronidazole and ampicillin. The erythema of rosacea sometimes responds to oral clonidine, and the flushing may be helped by a tranquillizer and avoidance of alcohol or heat.

Topical metronidazole is effective, and 1 per cent hydrocortisone cream, sulphur or ichthammol are also used. Potent topical steroids (p. 250) should be avoided in rosacea, as they present a special hazard. Patients are initially delighted with the response, and come back for repeat prescriptions but as time goes by their effect seems to decrease, and the redness and telangiectasia gradually become more marked. If the steroid application is reduced the condition deteriorates and more and more ointment is needed to maintain the 'status quo'. The patient has by this time become truly addicted to the steroid, since withholding the drug causes physical deterioration. Nevertheless, the only way to improve the erythema and atrophy is to stop the steroid, even though this produces a temporary

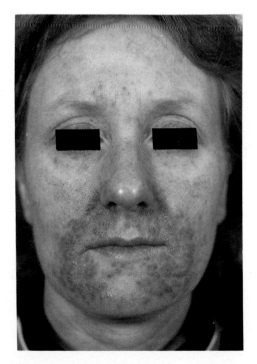

Fig. 5.7 Perioral dermatitis. A variant of rosacea

flare-up of the papules and pustules. Patients must be warned of this exacerbation, which may be modified by using a milder steroid ointment for a time.

The milder ocular complications of rosacea may be treated with oral oxytetracycline and steroid eye-drops, but keratitis demands the care of an ophthalmologist.

Rhinophyma does not respond to medical treatment, but surgical planing off of the surplus tissue gives amazingly good results.

Perioral dermatitis

This condition has become more common since the introduction of potent topical steroids. It tends to affect young women and it is characterized by erythema, papules and pustules around the mouth and naso-labial folds (Fig. 5.7). It is probably a variant of rosacea, and responds to the same treatment if topical steroids are avoided.

6

Disorders of sweat glands

There are two types of sweat glands in man, *eccrine* and *apocrine*. They differ in their distribution and in their pathology.

ECCRINE SWEAT GLANDS

These occur over virtually the whole body surface, but they are most profuse in the palms, soles and axillae. Sweat decreases the body temperature by evaporation, but it also helps to maintain the pliability of the keratin layer and to increase friction on the palms and soles. Some drugs such as alcohol are also excreted in the sweat.

Sweat is formed by a process of active secretion (the sodium pump) in the coils at the base of the gland, and its electrolyte composition is further modified as it travels up the intra-dermal portion of the sweat duct. The process is somewhat analagous to the formation of urine in the nephron, and some drugs (e.g., aldosterone and ADH) which affect the renal tubules also act on the sweat ducts. The terminal part of the duct pursues a corkscrew course through the epidermis and this arrangement helps to maintain its patency during changes in epidermal hydration.

Sweat contains sodium, potassium, chloride, lactate, urea and ammonia. Increased concentration of sodium chloride in sweat is found in fibrocystic disease (mucoviscidosis) and sweat chloride estimation is a helpful diagnostic test. Metal handled by certain workers in the light engineering industry tends to rust abnormally quickly and these workers ('rusters') also excrete more chloride in their sweat than their colleagues.

Sweat production is regulated by the sympathetic nervous system and the fibres to sweat glands are unusual in secreting acetylcholine rather than adrenaline i.e., they are cholinergic sympathetic fibres. There are three types of stimuli for sweating:

1. *Thermal* Sweating follows a rise in central core temperature (due to exercise or pyrexia) or a rise in ambient temperature. The

body 'thermostat' is in the hypothalamus, and pyrogens released from leucocytes e.g., during infection, can increase the setting.

2. *Emotional* Any type of mental stress will increase sweating from the palms, soles and axillae (the 'cold sweat' of the cheap novel), and this is the basis of the electro-physiological 'lie detector'. In clinical practice mental arithmetic may be used to provoke emotional sweating. Various forms of physical stress such as nausea or hypoglycaemia will also stimulate sweating.

3. *Gustatory* Certain spicy foods will provoke sweating of the face. The sweat glands excrete from 300 ml to 12 litres of fluid each day, but a further 200 ml diffuses directly through the horny layer and this is called the *transepidermal water loss*. The total daily water loss from the skin under basal conditions is therefore about 500 ml.

'Heat stroke'

During exercise in hot dry conditions the amount of water and solutes excreted from the skin exceeds that from the kidney, and this can result in serious dehydration and electrolyte depletion unless the subject can drink freely. After some hours, sweat gland fatigue occurs and the body temperature rises. The subject feels dry and hot, and there may be weakness, headache, confusion and collapse. The syndrome will be familiar to fans of French Foreign Legion films.

DISORDERS OF ECCRINE SWEAT GLANDS

Hyperhidrosis

Excessive sweating may be generalised or localized. Hyperhidrosis of the palms is most common in young women. It may be so severe that the hands drip water during emotional stress and feel like cold cod-fish. This is not only a social nuisance, for it impairs the performance of many jobs such as typing.

Hyperhidrosis of the feet causes a foul smell, discolours the shoes, and predisposes to eczema and fungal infection.

Axillary hyperhidrosis is mainly a social problem which increases body odour, and stains and rots the clothing.

In most cases no cause is found, although some patients with an anxious disposition may be helped by tranquillizers. Organic disease such as acromegaly, thyrotoxicosis and tuberculosis must be excluded, and an overt anxiety state may need psychiatric help.

Treatment of hyperhidrosis

1. *Topical applications.* 20 per cent aluminium chloride hexahydrate in alcohol is often effective. The patient should go to bed, rest quietly for $\frac{1}{2}$ hr, then wash and dry the affected areas and apply the lotion. Initially treatment is required every night, but the intervals between applications may be gradually increased. This preparation is very effective for axillary hyperhidrosis, though it often causes irritation if the area has been recently shaved.

Topical glutaraldehyde solution blocks the sweat ducts but may cause contact dermatitis.

Poldine methosulphate, an anticholinergic preparation, may also be useful. Systemic anticholinergic drugs are not worthwhile, as they produce troublesome side-effects (dry mouth and blurred vision) before they reduce sweating.

2. *Iontophoresis.* A direct current of low voltage can be used to introduce ionized drugs into the skin. Glycopyrronium bromide is an anticholinergic drug which produces improvement by this technique, but iontophoresis of tap-water will also reduce sweating since the current selectively damages and blocks the sweat ducts. This treatment is useful for palmar hyperhidrosis though many patients find it irksome to attend hospital at regular intervals.

3. *Surgery.* Axillary hyperhidrosis can be cured by excision and undercutting of the affected skin. The area of densest sweat gland activity must be first identified by staining with starch and iodine.

Cervical or lumbar sympathectomy will reduce hyperhidrosis of the palms or soles respectively, but the operation is not free from risk, and some patients develop compensatory hyperhidrosis of the trunk.

Hypohidrosis

Lack of sweat production is not readily noticed by patients, although they may complain of heat intolerance.

Causes of hypohidrosis

1. *Hypohidrotic ectodermal dysplasia* This is a rare congenital syndrome characterized by sparse sweat glands, defective peg-shaped teeth, thin eyebrows and scalp hair and a characteristic facies. Such patients are susceptible to heat stroke, and some of them also have atopic eczema.

2. *Neuropathy* Any lesion of the sympathetic tract (from the hypothalamus to the terminal sympathetic fibres) can produce hypohidrosis and the localization of the hypohidrosis may be of diagnostic help to the neurologist e.g., sometimes the level of a spinal cord tumour can be determined by running the finger up the back and noting the change in skin texture as an aid to identification of the dermatome root. Diabetic neuropathy and leprosy are other important causes of localized hypohidrosis, which can be demonstrated by provocative testing by heat, exercise or local injection of a cholinergic drug.

3. *Skin disease* Miliaria and psoriasis are associated with a decreased sweating in the affected skin. In patients with erythroderma from any cause, sweating is reduced and temperature regulation is defective (p. 235).

4. *Prematurity* Many premature babies do not sweat, even when pyrexial.

Miliaria ('Prickly heat')

Miliaria is due to sweat duct blockage caused by over-hydration of keratin in hot humid conditions. It produces pruritus, small vesicles, erythema and papules and the clinical picture varies according to the depth of the blockage in the epidermis. In tropical conditions patients become susceptible to 'heat stroke' and the sweat glands may remain non-functioning for some weeks after apparent recovery.

Prevention depends on measures to increase sweat evaporation, and topical antibiotics and ascorbic acid 1g daily may also help. Topical steroids reduce the irritation and rash. The best treatment is removal to a cooler climate, but if this is not possible a long motor-bike ride may help.

APOCRINE GLANDS

These occur in the axillae, and around the nipples and the anogenital region. They open into hair follicles, and part of their secretion is produced by the breaking off of the tip of the secretory cell cytoplasm. They become active at puberty, and 'body-odour' is due to bacterial decomposition of the apocrine secretions. In some animals the apocrine secretions are very important in marking out territorial areas and in olfactory sexual attraction. It has been suggested that such pheromones might have a subliminal effect on human sexual physiology since women who live together in institutions have been found to synchronize their periods. In monkeys a free fatty acid called copulin has been isolated from the vaginal secretions. When copulin is sprayed on to a decrepit old female the virile young males fight over her. If this can be added to perfumes it threatens to be the ultimate aphrodisiac.

Hidradenitis suppurativa (apocrine acne)

This is a chronic suppurative disease of the apocrine glands which causes multiple tender papules and pustules, with persistent sinuses, fibrosis and scarring. Bacterial swabs are often negative, and the response to antibiotics is poor. It is sometimes associated with acne vulgaris and it may be a type of cystic acne of the apocrine glands.

It is a disease which causes much misery and in severe cases surgical excision and skin grafting of the axillae or groins may be required.

SWEAT GLAND TUMOURS

Many types of apocrine and eccrine sweat gland tumours occur, but they are of little significance and carcinoma is rare.

Syringoma

This benign adenoma of eccrine sweat glands causes multiple skin-coloured papules around the eyes which are often mistaken for basal cell carcinomata.

7

Disorders of collagen, elastin and ground substance

The dermis is composed mainly of interweaving fibres of collagen, which give it strength, and a smaller quantity of elastin fibres, which provide elasticity. These fibres are embedded in a gel called the ground substance.

COLLAGEN

Collagen is the most important structural protein in the body, being present in large quantities in skin (70 per cent of dry weight), bone, tendon and cartilage. It also has an important supportive role in many other tissues such as blood vessels, cornea, glomeruli etc.

Defects in collagen synthesis are known to produce rare but important congenital syndromes, (p. 80), and collagen overproduction plays a pathogenetic role in such diverse systemic diseases as cirrhosis, pulmonary fibrosis and systemic sclerosis. Our increasing knowledge of the factors controlling collagen synthesis and degradation is likely to find widespread clinical application in the future.

Biosynthesis of collagen

The basic collagen molecule is composed of 3 polypeptide chains called α-chains which are coiled round each other to form a triple helix like the strands of a rope. The 3 chains are held together by hydrogen bonds and inter-molecular cross-links. This unusual conformation gives the molecule a rigid rod-like structure (Fig. 7.1). These polypeptide chains are composed mainly of relatively unusual amino-acids such as glycine, proline and lysine. Some proline and lysine residues become hydroxylated to form hydroxyproline and hydroxylysine respectively. A critical amount of hydroxyproline is essential to stablize the triple helical conformation. Ascorbic acid is a cofactor for the prolyl hydroxylase enzyme and patients with

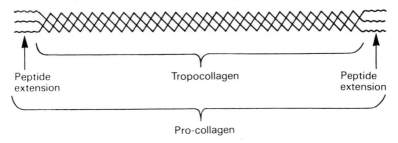

Fig. 7.1 Formation of collagen

scurvy have defective connective tissue and poor wound healing because they cannot form hydroxyproline.

There are several different types of collagen, each with different amino acid sequences, and they tend to occur in different tissues as follows:

Type I: Dermis, tendons and bones.

Type II: Cartilage.

Type III: Dermis and blood vessels.

Type IV: Basement membranes.

Collagen is initially synthesized in the fibroblasts as a larger precursor molecule called *procollagen*. After secretion from the cell, the procollagen molecules are converted to *tropocollagen* by peptidase enzymes which remove the peptide extensions at each end of the molecule by a process of limited proteolysis. A lack of these peptidases in some cattle causes the disease call *dermatosparaxis*, in which the skin and other tissues are extremely fragile. One type of Ehlers-Danlos syndrome in man may result from a similar defect, (p. 80).

After removal of the peptide extensions, the collagen molecules spontaneously align to form fibrils. The tropocollagen molecules, each composed of 3 α-chains, aggregate as shown, each with a stagger of a quarter of a molecular length, to form a fibril (Fig. 7.2).

These fibrils do not, however, attain their full tensile strength until the molecules are linked by covalent bonds called *cross-links*. The first step in the production of the cross-links is the formation of aldehydes from the lysyl and hydroxylysyl residues. This requires the enzyme lysyl oxidase, and its action is blocked by nitriles, which occur in some plants such as sweet peas. A sweet pea diet in cattle causes *lathyrism*, which is characterized by joint deformity and aortic aneurysm due to defective collagen. The levels

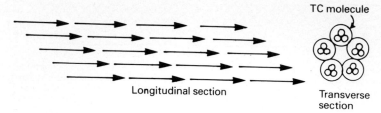

Fig. 7.2 Fibril of aggregated tropocollagen molecules

of lysyl oxidase are low in some patients with the Ehlers-Danlos syndrome.

The aldehydes then form two types of covalent cross-links, which may be either intra-molecular, between two adjacent α-chains, or inter-molecular, stabilizing the alignment of two neighbouring tropocollagen molecules in the fibril. This reaction, which is essential for the maturation and stability of collagen, is prevented by the drug penicillamine.

Degradation of collagen

The bulk of collagen in the body is metabolically active, and even the most stable fibres are slowly replaced by those newly synthesized. The degradation process is initiated by a specific enzyme called *collagenase*, but increased cross-linking of the collagen molecules decreases the rate of degradation. Collagenases are increased following parturition, when they are required for involution of the enlarged uterus. Recent work has suggested that increased collagenase activity may be important in some types of epidermolysis bullosa (p. 206). In the tadpole, thyroxine stimulates collagenase activity so that the large tail is resorbed as the tadpole matures into a frog.

Langer's lines

If the skin is punctured by a sharp circular spike, the wound gapes open due to the skin elasticity, but the hole is elliptical rather than circular. This is because the collagen fibres of the dermis when viewed from the skin surface form a network with a rhomboidal mesh (Fig. 7.3), and the skin therefore stretches more easily in some directions than others. The lines of least tension are called Langer's lines, and surgical scars heal quicker and give a better

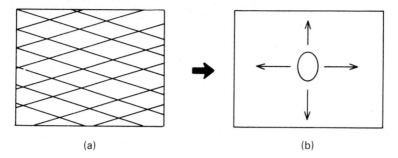

(a)   (b)

Fig. 7.3 (a) Orientation of the collagen fibres (b) Elliptical hole produced by a circular wound

cosmetic result if the incision is made along the lines rather than across them. This is most important on the face and neck, where the lines correspond roughly to the direction of the incipient wrinkles.

A. Diseases due to defective collagen

1. Solar elastosis

Damage to the skin by chronic exposure to ultra-violet radiation causes the formation of abnormal collagen which has many of the characteristics of elastin, with curling and fragmentation of the fibres. This is readily recognized clinically, since the skin becomes thickened, yellow and wrinkled, and on the neck the skin is furrowed into rhomboidal patterns. Solar elastosis occurs on the exposed parts, and is sometimes accompanied by a tendency to comedo formation.

The other characteristics of aged skin (fragility, easy bruising, loss of elasticity and wrinkling) are also due to changes in the connective tissue. From early adulthood onwards, there is a gradual decrease in skin collagen, even from the covered parts.

2. Striae ('Stretch marks')

These unsightly linear reddish-purple marks are due to tears in the dermal collagen. They occur when new collagen production cannot keep pace with a sudden growth of the underlying tissues. Thus they occur on the abdomen and breasts during pregnancy, and on the lower back or outer thighs of adolescents following a growth spurt.

Glucocorticoids cause atrophy of collagen, and so striae also develop in patients with Cushing's disease. They can also be due to systemic steroid therapy, or prolonged application of potent topical steroids, especially under polythene occlusion. There is no satisfactory treatment for striae but they fade and become inconspicuous as the years go by.

3. Ehlers-Danlos syndrome (Cutis hyperelastica)

This is a rare inherited disease characterized by various collagen defects and at least ten distinct types have so far been identified. Premature delivery of the baby due to ruptured membranes is common, and the baby is often 'floppy'. Later on, the skin becomes soft, velvety and hyperextensible, and the joints are hypermobile. Affected patients have in the past made a good living in side-shows as 'The Elastic Man' or as professional contortionists. The fragile skin tends to scar easily, bruising is common and some patients die of massive haemorrhage or dissected aorta due to the defective connective tissue in the vessels.

4. Thin skin with osteoporosis

The skin may be thin and 'transparent' in patients with osteoporosis, even when not related to steroid therapy, and this is thought to be due to a primary defect in collagen production.

5. Osteogenesis imperfecta

This rare disease is characterized by excessively fragile bones, thin skin, defective teeth, hypermobile joints, otosclerosis and blue sclerae. Some cases are due to failure of the fibroblasts to synthesize normal quantities of type 1 collagen.

B. Diseases associated with over-production of collagen

1. Keloids

In this condition the connective tissue response to skin damage is excessive so that a firm, raised, smooth, pink plaque is produced instead of a neat scar (Fig. 7.4). The trauma may be trivial, but the presence of infection or foreign material in a wound predisposes to keloid formation. Keloids tend to be familial, and are commoner in Negroes, but they rarely occur in infancy or during old age. Keloids will respond in the early stages to repeated intra-lesional injections of triamcinolone. Radiotherapy decreases keloid pro-

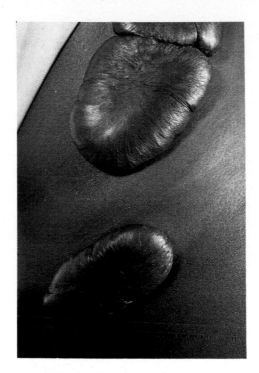

Fig. 7.4 Keloids which developed spontaneously

duction and some authorities advocate pre-operative radiation of the area if keloid formation is anticipated.

2. Plastic induration of the penis (Peyronie's disease)

In this rare but distressing disease of middle-aged men, a plaque of firm fibrous tissue develops in the penis, causing painful curvature during erection. This may be associated with Dupuytren's contracture of the palmar aponeurosis, and fibrous pads over the knuckles.

3. Scleroderma

This refers to sclerosis of the skin and subcutaneous tissue. Morphoea and systemic sclerosis are important causes (p. 222).

ELASTIN

This fibrillar material comprises only about 4 per cent of the dry skin weight. Its chemical composition is similar to that of collagen, but it is much more elastic. With increasing age the elastic tissue in the dermis degenerates, and the skin tends to sag and wrinkle. This seems to be a cause for universal concern, and the ability to rejuvenate dermal elastic tissue by the injection of the appropriate enzymes would be rather more lucrative than the ability to turn lead into gold.

Diseases due to defective elastin

1. Cutis laxa (Generalized elastolysis)

This is a rare disease, usually congenital, in which the elastic fibres are fragmented and disordered, so that the skin hangs in loose folds. This produces a facial appearance reminiscent of a blood-hound. The skin is easily stretched, but it does not spring back when released. The joints are not abnormal but pulmonary emphysema, herniae and large vessel defects occur.

2. Blepharochalasia

In this condition the skin around the eyes becomes lax and droopy, giving an appearance of world-weary debauchery. It is treated by plastic surgery.

3. Pseudo-xanthoma elasticum

This rare syndrome is characterized by distinctive skin lesions and grey angioid streaks in the retina. There is a tendency to massive haemorrhage, especially from the gastrointestinal tract because the elastic tissue of the blood vessels is abnormal. The skin is often loose and wrinkled around the neck and axillae, with small yellow-ish papules (resembling xanthomata) arranged linearly (Fig. 7.5).

In the early stages of the disease calcium is deposited on apparently normal elastic fibres, but these later become swollen and degenerate.

GROUND SUBSTANCE

This is composed of a complex mixture of acid mucopolysaccharides (glycosaminoglycans) and mucoproteins, and it probably regulates the transmission of hormones and nutrients from blood vessels to cells.

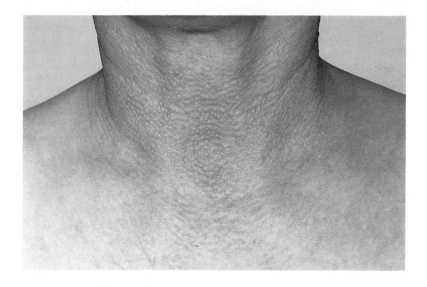

Fig. 7.5 Pseudo-xanthoma elasticum, showing the characteristic yellow tinge

Diseases associated with excessive ground substance

1. Myxoedema

This terms refers to accumulation of mucin in the dermis. Generalized myxoedema is a common feature of hypothyroidism, but pretibial myxoedema is a complication of hyperthyroidism, especially with raised levels of LATS (long-acting thyroid stimulator). Pretibial myxoedema produces raised, reddish-blue plaques over the shins, but the regular application of a potent topical steroid under polythene occlusion will cause considerable improvement.

2. Mucopolysaccharidoses

These are rare recessive genetic disorders characterized by excessive deposition of mucopolysaccharides in various tissues such as skin, joints and bones. There are at least six types, of which Hurler's syndrome (gargoylism) with dwarfism and mental deficiency is the best known. The basic abnormality may be a defect in the lysosomal enzymes which break down mucopolysaccharides.

8

Disorders of blood vessels and lymphatics

The skin has an abundant blood supply which is finely regulated over a wide range by the sympathetic nervous system in order to maintain the normal body temperature. Arterioles run upwards in the fibrous tissue septa of the subcutaneous fat, and then branch to form an intercommunicating plexus in the lower dermis. This supplies the various secreting glands, hair follicles etc. but some branches continue upwards to form a second plexus at the base of the papillae, from which capillary loops supply each dermal papilla (Fig. 8.1).

In the dermis of the hands and feet there are multiple small, richly innervated AV shunts called glomus bodies. Rarely one may become hyperplastic, to form a painful glomus tumour.

Lympatic vessels are also very abundant in the dermis but they are not normally seen in biopsy specimens as they are extremely thin-walled channels which collapse when the block is dehydrated.

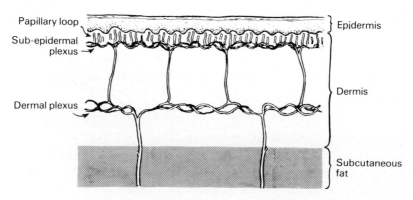

Fig. 8.1 Blood supply of skin

DISORDERS OF THE CIRCULATION

The blood vessels are involved in many diseases as a result of the release of vasoactive chemicals, and the classification of vascular disease is therefore somewhat arbitrary. Urticaria (p. 165), for example may be due to the pharmacological effects of certain drugs, or to an immunological defect, and yet it ultimately depends on a vascular response.

Erythema

Erythema, localized or widespread, is a feature of all inflammatory skin diseases.

Widespread erythema may be due to systemic viral or bacterial infection (e.g., rubella or scarlatina) or to a drug eruption. Often no definite cause can be found for a widespread urticated erythema, and this is then called a 'toxic erythema'.

Figurate erythema is a rare chronic disorder in which recurrent annular or figurate lesions slowly extend and fade over several weeks. It is sometimes due to underlying malignancy or hypersensitivity to a fungus, but often no cause is found.

Erythema of the palms occurs in pregnancy, and in liver disease, due to increased oestrogens (Fig. 8.2).

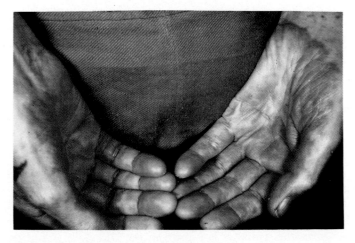

Fig. 8.2 Palmar erythema due to alcoholic cirrhosis

Flushing

Flushing is a transient diffuse vasodilatation of the face which often spreads to involve the neck and upper chest. It occurs in normal people as a result of heat, exercise or emotion ('blushing'). This is one of the commonest signs in medicine, since many women develop blotchy erythema of the neck and upper chest whenever they are examined.

Flushing is also commonly provoked by the ingestion of *alcohol* or *hot drinks*. In the latter case the flushing may be due to a counter-current heat exchange mechanism. The hot beverage inceases the temperature of the blood draining the oral cavity, and heat exchange between the internal jugular vein and the internal carotid artery may result in a slight increase in temperature in the hypothalamus, which responds by provoking heat-dissipating reactions such as sweating and flushing. The active agent in hot coffee which causes flushing is heat, not caffeine.

The exact mechanism of alcohol-induced flushing is uncertain, though it is probably related to increased blood acetaldehyde levels. There has been great interest recently in the flushing reaction which develops in some diabetic patients who drink alcohol after taking *chlorpropamide*. The reaction is similar to that which occurs in normal subjects who take alcohol after disulfiram. It is thought that endogenous opioids, such as enkephalin, play a role in the production of chlorpropamide-ethanol flushing, and possibly also in the pathogenesis of alcoholism.

Flushing is a common feature of *rosacea*, especially after the ingestion of hot drinks or alcohol, and some authors believe this is one of the main factors in the pathogenesis of the disease (p. 66).

Paroxysmal flushing is common at the *menopause*. The flushing is accompanied by the pulsatile release of luteinizing hormone from the pituitary, though this hormone is not the cause of the flush, since it can occur even after hypophysectomy. It seems likely that a neuronal discharge from the hypothalamus spreads to the nearby temperature regulating centre, and re-sets the thermostat so that the poor afflicted lady suddenly exclaims 'Isn't it hot in here?' as she sweats, flushes and rushes around throwing open all the windows to let in the snow. Both the luteinizing hormone release and the antisocial behaviour can be prevented by replacement oestrogen therapy. Incidentally, the feeling which provokes the antisocial urge to fling open the windows is known in the U.S.A. as a 'hot flash', whereas British 'flashers' exhibit quite different antisocial behaviour.

Systemic diseases which are associated with flushing include the dumping syndrome and various forms of malignancy, in which the vasodilatation is probably related to prostaglandin release. The association of flushing with asthma and diarrhoea should suggest the possibility of a carcinoid tumour. Sometimes an attack can be provoked by abdominal palpation, since carcinoid tumours occur most commonly in the appendix. The association of flushing with paroxysmal hypertension (as suggested by a history of transient throbbing headaches for example) may be due to a phaeochromocytoma.

Many other reactions are known to bring a flush to the cheeks, including the 'Chinese restaurant syndrome', in which flushing and asthma result from ingestion of monosodium glutamate. Flushing can also be due to drugs such as calcium channel blockers (nifedipine, verapamil, etc.) and vasodilators (e.g., amyl nitrite inhaled for 'recreational' purposes). Maidenly blushes are now virtually unknown.

Telangiectases

These are permanently dilated small vessels. They occur commonly in cutaneous atrophy from any cause, e.g., ageing, radiation, application of steroid ointments, etc. Venous hypertension (p. 90) often causes a leash of telangiectatic vessels around the ankle, and nail fold capillary telangiectases are a useful sign of collagen-vascular disease.

'Spider' telangiectases

The name derives from the dilated capillaries which radiate like spider legs from the central arteriole. Isolated 'spiders' are common in normal people, but they often increase in number during pregnancy or in liver disease. A good cosmetic result can be produced by cauterization of the central feeding vessel.

Hereditary haemorrhagic telangiectasia

This is a dominant genetic disorder which usually presents with epistaxis or gastro-intestinal haemorrhage. It should be recognized by Casualty Officers by the small red spots on the lips and tongue which blanch on pressure (Fig. 8.3). Recurrent epistaxes may be a problem despite cauterization, and oestrogens sometimes help these patients, probably by increasing keratinization of the nasal mucosa. Iron supplements are also required.

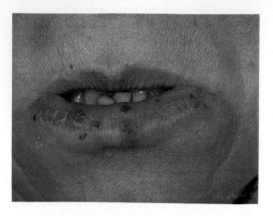

Fig. 8.3 Hereditary haemorrhagic telangiectasia

Urticaria and vasculitis (see Chapter 15)

Purpura

Extravasation of red blood cells has many causes, and these may be simply classified as disorders of platelets, vessels or coagulation.

Disorders of platelets and coagulation tend to produce ecchymoses and external bleeding, and most purpura seen in dermatological practice is due to vascular changes. Many inflammatory dermatoses such as eczema can produce purpura, especially at sites of venous hypertension (e.g., the ankle), but there are many other causes including vasculitis, senility, drugs (e.g., carbromal or topical steroids), infections (e.g., meningococcaemia), dysproteinaemia, etc.

There are also several chronic purpuric dermatoses of unknown cause, the names of which (e.g., 'pigmented purpuric lichenoid dermatosis of Gougerot and Blum') cause more trouble to the patient than the disease itself.

Perniosis ('chilblains')

Chilblains are localized inflammatory lesions which are provoked by exposure to cold. They occur on the fingers, feet or ears, as reddish-blue swellings which are characteristically painful or itchy on rewarming after exposure to cold. The pathogenesis is uncertain, but prolonged vasoconstriction of venules appears to be important. The disease is most common in obese young women, especially those who stand on wind-swept streets in Northern winters, waiting for buses or boyfriends which never arrive.

The treatment of chilblains is unsatisfactory, but warm housing, warm clothing and erythema doses of UVR may be prophylactic. Vasodilators are of very limited value but severe cases may respond to sympathectomy.

Livedo reticularis

This is a reticulate cyanosis with a 'mesh' of 1–4 cm in diameter. The abnormal bluish-red areas of the network correspond to areas where the capillaries dilate and the blood flow stagnates.

It is a physiological response to cold in children, but in older people the change suggests the possibility of underlying arterial disease (e.g., atheroma or vasculitis) especially if the change is patchy ('broken livedo').

Erythema ab igne

This is a reticulate pigmented erythema, often with slight scaling, which is due to chronic infra-red radiation. The pattern is similar to livedo reticularis. It usually follows 'toasting the legs' before a coal-fire, or constantly clutching a hot-water bottle to the site of some intractable pain. It is a degenerative change which is occasionally premalignant.

Raynaud's phenomenon

This is a paroxysmal constriction of the digital vessels which causes a sequence of colour changes — pallor (due to ischaemia), cyanosis (due to dilated capillaries with stagnant blood flow) and then erythema (due to reactive hyperaemia). Attacks are usually precipitated by cold, or by carrying heavy shopping bags. There are many causes, including:

(i)   Collagen vascular disease, especially systemic sclerosis
(ii)   Arterial occlusion, e.g., thoracic outlet syndromes, atheroma, Buerger's disease, etc.
(iii) Reflux vasoconstriction due to occupational trauma (e.g., typing, pneumatic drilling), or other injury.
(iv)   Increased blood viscosity e.g., dysproteinaemia
(v)   Neurological disease, e.g., syringomyelia or paralysis
(vi)   Toxins, e.g., heavy metals, ergot, vinyl chloride

The term Raynaud's *disease* refers to Raynaud's phenomenon for which no cause is found. Most cases have a good prognosis, but it must be remembered that Raynaud's phenomenon can be the presenting feature of systemic sclerosis for some years before the other symptoms develop.

Venous hypertension of the legs (the 'gravitational' syndrome)

The venous drainage of the legs depends upon three sets of veins, the deep veins (surrounded by muscles), the superficial veins, and the numerous communicating veins which connect the other two systems. The blood is pumped back to the heart against gravity only if the leg muscles are active, and the valves in the veins are intact. Pump failure leads to increased hydrostatic pressure in the venules, particularly on standing, and this in turn causes leakage of plasma through the endothelial pores of the capillaries. This forms a layer of peri-capillary fibrin which interferes with the transfer of blood gases and metabolites. The old term 'venous stasis' should not be applied to this condition, since the blood flow to the affected skin is actually increased.

Venous insufficiency is usually caused by obstruction of the deep veins by thrombosis, or by valvular destruction by a previous thrombosis. This may have occurred after childbirth, surgical operations, injury to the leg (especially fractures) or prolonged bed rest and often the patient is unaware that thrombosis has occurred. Constipation due to a low fibre diet may also play a part in causing venous hypertension, since the condition is rare in communities which have a high fibre diet and a rapid colonic transit time.

The clinical features of the 'gravitational' syndrome are:

(i) *Varicose veins* These are tortuous dilatations of the superficial veins, and though they are caused by venous insufficiency, they are not an essential part of the syndrome.

(ii) *Oedema* Chronic accumulation of tissue fluid may eventually lead to induration and fibrosis of the tissue around the ankle, which further limits the action of the calf muscle pump.

(iii) *Eczema* Redness, scaling and irritation are common, and the explanation for this is unknown. The condition can be very severe, and there may be 'secondary spread' to other parts of the body (p. 178).

(iv) *Pigmentation* There may be post-inflammatory hypermelanosis in addition to haemosiderin deposits derived from red cells extravasated by the increased capillary pressure.

(v) *Atrophie blanche* This is a white plaque of sclerosis, stippled with telangiectases, and often surrounded by hyperpigmentation.

(vi) *Ulceration* This characteristically develops just above the medial malleolus, following mild trauma. The ulcer slowly enlarges and because of the insidious progression, patients are often slow to seek medical advice. Secondary infection is common.

Treatment of ulceration secondary to venous hypertension

The primary aim should be to reduce venous hypertension by compressive bandages so that natural healing will occur. A paste bandage covered by an elastic adhesive is usually most satisfactory, but the particular preparation used is far less important than the skill of the nurse who applies it. Patients shouuld be encouraged to walk (but not stand) with the bandage on, since this increases arterial blood flow, improves the muscle pump, and prevents the deep vein thrombosis and contractures which so readily develop in elderly recumbent patients. In a clean granulating ulcer the dressing needs to be changed only once or twice weekly. Any bland local antiseptic preparation such as 50 per cent Eusol in paraffin emulsion may be used to clean the ulcer. Secondary infection must be treated, by systemic antibiotics if necessary, but some organisms isolated from leg ulcers may be 'passengers' which cause little trouble. The possibility of sensitization to topical antibiotics or ointment bases must be constantly borne in mind.

Weight reduction should be attempted in the obese, and correction of any deficiency of iron, ascorbic acid or folate is essential. Zinc deficiency retards wound healing, but double-blind trials of oral zinc therapy have shown no benefit in venous leg ulcers.

Firm sloughs may prevent re-epithelialization, and these may be cleared by a proteolytic preparation such as malic acid provided the surrounding skin is protected.

Large ulcers which have granulated can be re-epithelialized more quickly by the application of multiple small skin grafts taken from the thigh.

Once the ulcer has healed, patients should continue to wear elastic stockings and should protect the vulnerable area from further trauma by a gauze pad. Surgical treatment such as injection of perforating veins should be considered for suitable patients, but long-term follow-up shows that surgery is often unsuccessful in preventing recurrent ulceration.

Other causes of leg ulcers

Though venous hypertension is by far the commonest cause of leg ulcers, it is not the only cause. The following possibilities should be considered, particularly if other signs of the 'gravitational syndrome' are absent, or if the ulcer is in an unusual site.

1. Ischaemia

In severe atheroma the foot pulses will be absent or greatly diminished. The toes will be cold and blue, and pressure on the ischaemic skin produces prolonged blanching. The ulcer is often painful, but the pain is sometimes helped by dangling the leg over the side of the bed, so that gravity helps the arterial blood flow. There may or may not be a history of intermittent claudication.

Ulcers due to vasculitis often have an irregular margin and a 'punched-out' edge, unlike the gently shelving edge of venous ulcers.

2. Neuropathy (e.g., diabetes, spina bifida)

3. Rheumatoid disease (p. 224)

4. Malignancy

In squamous cell carcinoma the base of the ulcer is indurated.

5. Rare causes These include haemolytic anaemia (especially sickle-cell disease), gumma, necrobiosis lipoidica (p. 226), pyoderma gangrenosum (p. 213) and hypertension.

Leg ulcers in old people often have several causes, e.g., venous hypertension, atheroma, anaemia and infection.

LYMPHOEDEMA

Oedema due to inadequate lymphatic drainage is often firm and non-pitting due to organization and fibrosis, and the overlying epidermis may become grossly hyperkeratotic. Lymphoedema may be *primary*, due to a developmental defect in the lymphatics, or *secondary* to some other pathology such as malignant infiltration, surgical destruction, irradiation, filariasis (p. 144) or recurrent lymphangitis.

Lymphangiography following injection of radio-opaque material into a small peripheral lymphatic may help to localize the site of blockage.

Treatment of lymphoedema

This is unsatisfactory, but diuretics and pressure bandages may help. Various reconstructive surgical procedures may be tried in severe cases. Lymphoedema seems to predispose to episodes of recurrent infection with haemolytic streptococci and these attacks of erysipelas often cause further damage to the lymphatics, so that a vicious circle occurs. Long-term penicillin therapy may help these cases.

9

Tumours and naevi

A cutaneous naevus is a circumscribed developmental anomaly of the skin, and though naevi are often present at birth (i.e., true 'birth-marks'), others do not become apparent until adult life. They may continue to proliferate after birth so that the distinction between a naevus and a benign neoplasm is not always clear, and some naevi tend to undergo malignant degeneration in later life.

A neoplasm may be benign or malignant, but in some cutaneous lesions, such as the *kerato-acanthoma* (p. 105), the distinction is not clear-cut, since the histology may look malignant, but the condition may resolve spontaneously. In general, benign skin tumours present as slowly-growing nodules, whereas the malignant ones present in a variety of forms, with or without ulceration, ranging from slowly-growing nodules to more aggressive forms which grow rapidly and metastasize early.

A. MALIGNANT NEOPLASIA ARISING FROM EPIDERMIS

The commonest three skin malignancies are the *squamous cell carcinoma*, which arises from keratinizing epidermis, the *basal cell carcinoma* which probably arises from the hair follicle epithelium, and the *malignant melanoma* which originates from the melanocyte.

Predisposing factors

1. Radiation

Ultra-violet irradiation of the skin is the most important cause of epidermal malignancy. Both squamous carcinoma and basal cell carcinoma are much commoner in light exposed parts of the body, and their incidence increases with advancing age since the damage caused by UVR is cumulative. UVR also predisposes to malignant melanoma, but the relationship is less clearly defined since the lesion often arises on the covered skin in young people.

All three neoplasia are more common in places such as Florida and Australia which have much sunshine, and a population of white people striving to become brown. Naturally dark-skinned people are resistant to UVR-induced damage, but those with a 'Celtic complexion' (p. 27) are particularly prone to develop degenerative changes and malignancy in later life. Albinos, because of their lack of protective melanin are also at particular risk and albinos working outdoors in the tropics frequently die in their twenties from multiple skin malignancies.

The incidence of skin cancer, particularly malignant melanoma, is currently rising sharply in the Western world, and this is partly due to the increased availability of cheap 'package' holidays, which offer a tempting combination of sun, sea, see and sin. Most young people who indulge in such holidays realize the risk of diarrhoea, gonorrhoea and amenorrhoea, but few of them worry about the risk of skin cancer, which may develop 30 years later.

X-rays in high dosage cause 'radiation dermatitis', which is a premalignant condition. It is characterized by pigmentation, atrophy and telangiectasia in the irradiated area.

Chronic infra-red irradiation causes 'erythema ab igne' (p. 89), and this may also undergo malignant degeneration.

2. Chemicals

Some chemicals such as benzpyrene which is present in car and aircraft exhaust fumes are undoubtedly carcinogenic when repeatedly applied to mouse skin, but their role in causing human skin cancer is unknown. Chemical carcinogens such as tar, pitch and mineral oil have in the past caused occupational skin cancers in chimney sweeps, shale oil workers, cotton mill spinners, etc. Arsenic is also carcinogenic (p. 232).

3. Scars

Malignancy occasionally arises in old scars, particularly those due to severe burns or lupus vulgaris.

4. Immune responses

The concept of 'immune surveillance' suggests that some malignant cells are destroyed by the body's immune defence mechanisms soon after they arise. Immune deficiency might therefore predispose to malignancy. Patients with multiple solar keratoses (p. 159) who have received immunosuppressive drugs after renal transplantation have a greatly increased incidence of skin cancer. It has recently been shown that ultra-violet radiation diminishes the immune responses, and this effect may be important in provoking cutaneous malignancy.

5. Genetic

A few rare congenital diseases predispose to cutaneous malignancy. They are important because they may help our understanding of carcinogenesis.

Xeroderma pigmentosum is one such disease, in which multiple cutaneous keratoses and malignancies develop during childhood. The cells in these patients are unable to perform the enzymatic 'repair-replication' of DNA which occurs in normal people following sunburn damage to nuclear material. Presumably this causes cumulative defects in epidermal DNA which predispose to malignant mitoses.

1. Squamous cell carcinoma

This usually arises in light-exposed areas of skin showing signs of chronic damage from UV irradiation, e.g., solar keratoses, elastotic degeneration, irregular pigmentation and telangiectasia (p. 159). Squamous carcinoma may form a flat plaque or a papule, and the surface may be keratotic or ulcerated, but in most cases the lesion is characteristically indurated on palpation. On the lip the presenting feature is usually a small ulcer which fails to heal and bleeds recurrently. Squamous carcinomata grow relatively slowly and they metastasize only at a late stage.

The histology shows a grossly disorganized epidermis, with hyperkeratosis, parakeratosis, frequent mitotic figures, and invasion of the dermis by strands of abnormal keratinocytes.

Bowen's disease is an intra-epidermal carcinoma which has not yet become invasive. Clinically it produces a persistent red scaly plaque which may be mistaken for psoriasis (Fig. 9.1). The histology is characteristic, with loss of epidermal polarity, many large atypical cells and frequent mitotic figures, but few lesions become frankly malignant.

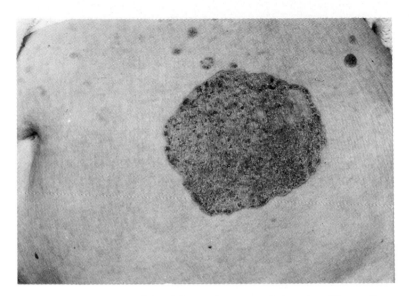

Fig. 9.1 Bowen's disease of the abdomen due to arsenic ingestion. The smaller
lesions are seborrhoeic warts

2. Basal cell carcinoma

This is the commonest skin malignancy, and the face is the commonest site to be affected. The early lesion is a small pearly pink
papule, often with a few overlying telangiectases. At a later stage
the epidermis breaks down to form an ulcer with a characteristic
rolled edge ('rodent ulcer'). Untreated lesions will slowly erode the
underlying tissues such as cartilage (Fig. 9.2), bone, brain or blood-
vessels but they hardly ever metastasize. Basal cell carcinoma occasionally presents in other forms e.g., as pigmented lesions, large
domed papules or flat indurated plaques (Fig. 9.3), which are often
misdiagnosed.

Treatment of squamous cell and basal cell carcinoma

These tumours may be treated either by

1. Local destruction, e.g., cauterization and curettage
2. Radiotherapy
3. Surgical excision

The choice depends on the size and site of the tumour and the
age of the patient. Some areas such as the dorsum of the hand

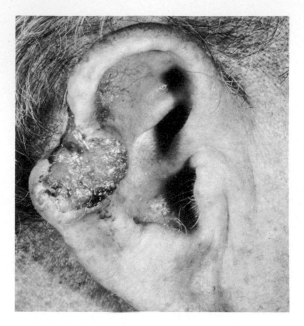

Fig. 9.2 Cartilage erosion by a basal cell cancer

should not be treated by radiotherapy because of the fragile scars produced. Small well-differentiated squamous lesions are best treated with local destruction or excision, whereas radiotherapy is more suitable for large, poorly differentiated lesions of the face. The five year cure rate in several large series has exceeded 95 per cent.

3. Malignant melanoma

This may arise in a pre-existing melanocytic naevus (p. 108) but about half the cases arise in skin which has previously appeared normal. Signs of possible malignancy in a pigmented lesion include enlargement, change in colour (whether darker or lighter), bleeding or ulceration, itching, inflammation or spread of pigment beyond the edge of the lesion. Most malignant melanomata are pigmented, but they occasionally present as a red fleshy papule, the 'amelanotic melanoma'.

There are three main types of malignant melanoma:

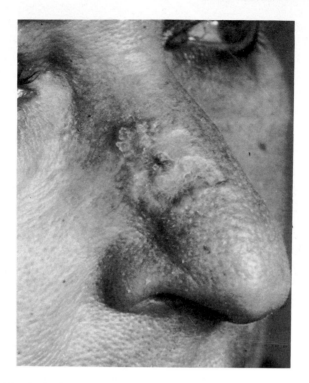

Fig. 9.3 Morphoeic (fibrosing) basal cell cancer. The 'rolled edge' is a diagnostic clue

1. Superficial spreading melanoma

In this type the lession spreads laterally within the epidermis for some months before it invades the dermis. The prognosis for lesions of this type is relatively good, provided they are excised before ulceration or nodules have developed.

2. Nodular melanoma

This is a more aggressive type which readily ulcerates. It invades the dermis and metastasizes at an early stage.

3. Lentigo maligna melanoma

This is a relatively benign form of melanoma which develops in an irregular patch of pigmentation called a lentigo maligna (Hutchinson's freckle). These flat lesions, which are quite common on the face of elderly people, represent an *in situ* phase of the neoplasm which may persist for years or even decades without progressing, but eventually the development of a papule will indicate that the melanoma has started to invade the dermis. Although metastasis can occur, it is much less common than in the previous two types of melanoma. Treatment is not usually necessary until a papule develops, but the flat lesions can if necessary be frozen with liquid nitrogen for cosmetic reasons.

The course of malignant melanoma is unpredictable. Some lesions metastasize at a very early stage, but in general the incidence of metastases correlates with the depth of invasion of the primary tumour at excision. Melanomata are notorious for their tendency to produce the first clinical evidence of metastasis some 10 or more years after an apparently adequate operation. Malignant melanoma sometimes produces a brisk lymphocytic reaction and spontaneous resolution in such cases has been recorded. Much work has been done on the immunotherapy of malignancy by BCG inoculation etc. but the practical applications are still very limited.

Treatment

Malignant melanoma must be completely excised as early as possible, including a margin of 'normal' skin around the edges. The pathologist should measure the tumour thickness in millimetres, and this will help the clinician to decide on further management. Lesions which are shown on histology to be less than 1 mm thick have a good 5-year survival rate (more than 90 per cent) following simple excision, but for thicker tumours, recurrence becomes more likely, and a wider excision with a skin graft will be required. The 5-year survival rate for tumours exceeding 3.5 mm in thickness is around 40 per cent and with distant metastases it is only 5 per cent. The effect of further treatment such as block dissection of the regional lymph nodes, chemotherapy and immunotherapy is controversial.

The clinical diagnosis of malignant melanoma is often difficult, even for the specialist. Many benign pigmented tumours masquerade as melanomata and they may provoke unnecessary mutilating surgery. The converse also applies, and malignant melanoma have often been inadvertently treated by curettage, with subsequent haematogenous dissemination. It is traditional to teach that a small incisional biopsy (as opposed to complete excision *ab inito*) predisposes to premature metastatic spread but the evidence for this is not good, and some authorities now believe that this procedure is safe provided that complete removal can be performed within the next few days.

B. OTHER CUTANEOUS MALIGNANCIES

1. Metastases

Small, hard cutaneous metastases are common in the terminal stages of systemic cancer. They may occasionally be the presenting manifestation, especially in the case of hypernephroma, which is often clinically silent and tends to metastasize to the scalp as a solitary vascular papule.

2. Cutaneous lymphoma

(i) Systemic malignant lymphomata such as Hodgkin's disease commonly cause non-specific cutaneous symptoms such as generalized pigmentation, pruritus or ichthyosis. Occasionally the lymphoma cells invade the skin directly to produce red papules or nodules, and lymphoma is a rare cause of erythroderma.

(ii) *Mycosis fungoides* is a T-cell lymphoma which arises *de novo* in the skin. Its exact pathogenesis is obscure, but it seems to start as chronic reactive lymphocytic infiltrate in the skin which after some years becomes truly malignant and eventually involves the systemic lymph nodes. In some cases a C-type retrovirus has been isolated from the skin lesions, but the significance of this is uncertain.

The disease usually starts in middle life, either as a non-specific red scaly rash (Fig. 9.4), or as a specific pre-myocotic eruption called *poikiloderma atrophicans vasculare*. This is characterized clinically by the appearance of red patches accompanied by reticulate pigmentation, telangiectasia and atrophy. The condition progresses slowly over 10 or 20 years, and the patches eventually assume a darker colour and become firmer. A biopsy at this stage may still be non-specific or it may reveal definite evidence of a malignant lymphoma. In many cases serial biopsies are required at intervals of months or years from several different sites. There is often increasing pruritus in the later stages. Eventually bluish-purple tumours develop in the skin (Fig. 9.5) and if untreated these ulcerate and discharge a foul fluid.

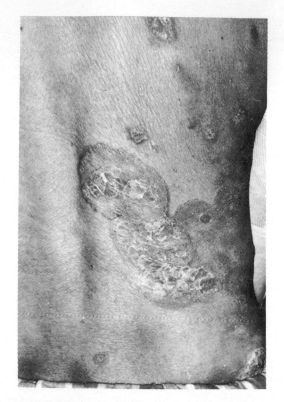

Fig. 9.4 Cutaneous lymphoma mimicking psoriasis

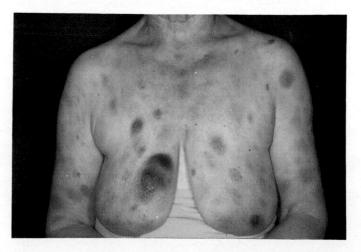

Fig. 9.5 Cutaneous lymphoma, showing the characteristic bluish colour

The histology of fully-developed mycosis fungoides shows a dense infiltrate in the superficial dermis, which tends to invade the epidermis to produce small micro-abscesses. Immature cells are seen, including the *mycosis cell* (Sézary cell), which is derived by blast transformation from a lymphocyte and which can be seen on electron miscroscopy to have a characteristic cerebriform nucleus (Fig. 9.6).

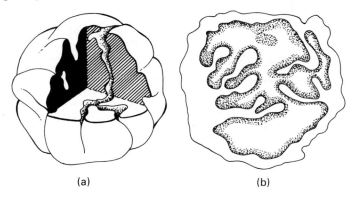

(a)   (b)

Fig. 9.6 The Sézary cell (a) Diagram of the cerebriform nucleus with a segment removed to show the convoluted profile. (b) The cell as it appears by electron microscopy

The Sézary syndrome is a variant of mycosis fungoides in which there is generalized pruritus, erythroderma and oedema, with large numbers of mycosis cells in the circulating blood. Some of these cases have probably been mistaken in the past for chronic lymphatic leukaemia.

Treatment of mycosis fungoides

In the early stages the condition may be kept in check by the application of a steroid ointment, and some cases will survive for 20 years or more before intensive treatment is required. In the later stages there are many lines of attack, including PUVA therapy, localized radiotherapy, whole-body electron beam therapy, topical application of nitrogen mustard and systemic cytotoxic drugs.

3. Leukaemia

In addition to the non-specific cutaneous markers of malignancy (p. 231), leukaemia may present with haemorrhage into the skin, erythroderma or with small pink papules which on biopsy are found to be crammed with immature white cells.

4. Paget's disease of the nipple

This is red, scaly, well-demarcated but slowly-spreading lesion of the nipple which is due to invasion of the epidermis by Paget cells from an underlying intra-duct carcinoma of the breast. Eczema of the areola may be mistaken for Paget's disease and a skin biopsy should be performed before mastectomy is undertaken. *Extra-mammary Paget's disease* may involve the ano-genital area, due to an underlying sweat-gland carcinoma, but this is rare.

5. Kaposi's sarcoma

Until a few years ago this vascular tumour was rarely seen outside Africa, but it has now achieved notoriety throughout the Western world as one of the manifestations of AIDS (the acquired immune deficiency syndrome), which occurs in sexually active homosexuals, heroin addicts, Haitians and haemophiliacs receiving pooled blood products. The tumour presents as one or more reddish-purple papules or nodules which on biopsy show proliferating capillaries with malignant spindle cells. A search for opportunistic infections, such as *Pneumocystis carinii* pneumonia, and full immunological investigations are required in any patient with Kaposi's sarcoma. In a patient with AIDS the prognosis is poor but, in the absence of AIDS, the speed of spread of the tumour is very variable, and excision or radiotherapy may produce a prolonged remission, though eventual recurrence is the rule.

BENIGN 'TUMOURS' AND CYSTS

1. 'Seborrhoeic' wart (basal cell papilloma)

The Lord Privy Seal is neither a lord, nor a privy, nor a seal, and 'seborrhoeic' warts have no relationship to seborrhoea. They are in fact masses of basaloid cells arranged in an orderly fashion, with overlying hyperkeratosis, and increased melanin production. The cause is unknown.

They are common in people over the age of 40, and are usually easy to recognize clinically. The lesions are fawn, brown or black papules which sometimes look greasy and they have a characteristic network of indentations or crypts on the surface. They are usually flattened, with an abrupt edge which is reminiscent of a blob of plasticine stuck on to the skin surface. They may be single or multiple, and the trunk and temples are the commonest sites. Occasionally they become inflamed, and are then easily mistaken for malignant melanoma.

Seborrhoeic warts do not become malignant, and they are easily removed by curettage or freezing with liquid nitrogen. Middle-aged ladies are the most likely to seek treatment, and the physician who describes the lesion by its alternative name of 'senile wart' is likely to be rewarded by a clout from a handbag.

2. Fibro-epithelial polyps and skin tags

A fibro-epithelial polyp is a pedunculated papule consisting of normal epidermis with a loose connective tissue stroma. Skin tags are small fibro-epithelial polyps. They are common in the elderly, often in association with seborrhoeic warts. They are particularly common on the neck and around the axillary folds. They can be cauterized or treated with liquid nitrogen.

3. Campbell de Morgan spots

These small bright red spots, due to capillary proliferation, occur on the trunk of most elderly patients. Their aetiology is unknown, and Final MB. examiners use them to fail really hopeless candidates.

4. Squamous papilloma and cutaneous horn

A squamous papilloma is a benign tumour arising from keratinocytes. It resembles a viral wart but can be distinguished from it histologically by the absence of viral inclusion bodies. In some cases the keratin production becomes excessive and a hard horn-shaped excrescence is produced. These are easily removed with a currette, but the base should be lightly cauterized, as they are sometimes premalignant.

5. Kerato-acanthoma

This is a fascinating lesion which looks malignant and acts benign. It grows rapidly for about six weeks to produce a large, indurated dome-shaped papule with a characteristic central crater filled by a keratinous plug (Fig. 9.7). The histology is often indistinguishable from squamous carcinoma, but it involutes spontaneously leaving a depressed scar. It is best to currette off the lesion and cauterize the base, since very rarely it may metastasize.

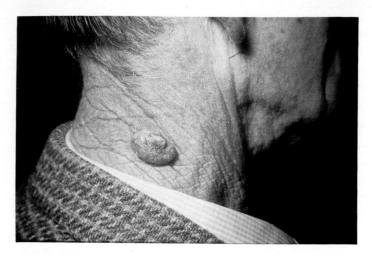

Fig. 9.7 Kerato-acanthoma

6. Lipoma

A lipoma is a fat cell tumour in the lower dermis or subcutaneous tissue. It is characteristically soft and lobulated on palpation. Occasionally there is an angiomatous component (angio-lipoma) and this type be tender or spontaneously painful. It is cured by excision.

7. Pyogenic granuloma

This is a soft, red, fleshy tumour which bleeds profusely when knocked. The finger is a common site. The histology shows many small capillaries with plump endothelial cells, surrounded by a mixed population of white cells. Most cases probably develop as a reactive change to a prick from a needle or a thorn.

8. Sclerosing haemangioma (histiocytoma, dermatofibroma)

These three names are attached to a very common but trivial lesion which is probably a reaction to trauma such as an insect bite. It presents as a single small skin-coloured nodule, usually on the lower leg. The histology shows either a mass of new capillaries, histiocytes or dense fibrous tissue, according to its stage of development.

9. Epidermoid cyst ('wen')

Many surgeons call this a 'sebaceous cyst' but in fact it is derived either from keratinizing epidermis or from hair follicle epithelium. The lesion presents as a smooth mobile lump, often on the scalp, and excision is simple and satisfying.

10. Milium

A milium is a small subepidermal keratin cyst. It produces a small white papule which rarely exceeds 2 mm in diameter. Milia are common on the face at all ages from infancy onward. In the adult they are easily expressed after incising the overlying epidermis with a cutting-edge needle.

11. Dermatosis papulosa nigra

This is a fairly common condition in which multiple, soft, small black papules develop on the cheeks of Negroes. Histologically they resemble seborrhoeic warts, but they start at a much earlier age, often at puberty.

12. Chondrodermatitis nodularis chronica helicis

It was probably a name like this which inspired the jibe that dermatologists are 'a priesthood mumbling a litany at the foot of a vague shrine.' The name refers to a painful firm papule on the helix of the ear which is the result of an inflammatory hyperkeratotic reaction around an area of damaged cartilage. It can be treated by currettage.

Many other benign skin tumours exist, some with endearing histological features and quaint names (e.g., calcifying epithelioma of Malherbe), but most of them present to the clinician as uninspiring single nodules. The more spectacular lesions, such as the 'turban tumour' of the scalp, are rare.

NAEVI

The common naevi such as 'moles' (which occur in over 95 per cent of white adults) are usually not associated with systemic developmental defects, but many inherited systemic diseases such as tuberous sclerosis and neurofibromatosis include cutaneous naevi as part of the syndrome.

Naevi often involve several cell types, but they may be classified according to their predominant component.

1. Melanocytic naevus ('Mole')

Melanocytes are derived from the neural crest, and they migrate through the mesoderm in the fetus to reach the epidermal basal layer. A 'mole' is a developmental defect which causes benign localized proliferation of melanocytes in the dermis. There may be associated abnormalities at the site of the naevus, such as large distorted hair follicles (Fig. 9.8) and a hyperkeratotic epidermis.

Histologically the abnormal melanocytes may occur:

(i)   At the epidermo-dermal junction only ('junctional' naevus)
(ii) As 'nests' of cells in the dermis ('intra-dermal' naevus)
(iii) At both sites ('compound' naevus).

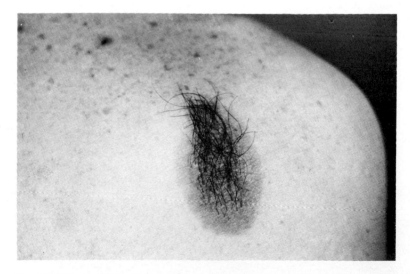

Fig. 9.8 Hairy melanocytic naevus

The lesion may not be apparent at birth, but may develop only in later life, especially at puberty or during pregnancy. As the patient matures the junctional cells tend to 'drop' into the dermis.

Melanocytic naevi vary considerably in size and appearance. They may be pink, brown or black, flat or raised, hairy or hairless, rough or smooth. They are potentially premalignant, but fortunately only a very small proportion actually undergo malignant change. Extensive, deeply pigmented, hairy naevi (Fig. 9.9) which are present at birth seem more likely to become malignant and should be treated by dermabrasion as soon after birth as possible.

Most 'moles' require no treatment, but suspect lesions (p. 98) should be excised for histological examination. They may also be removed for cosmetic reasons, or because of recurrent trauma from belts, etc.

Dysplastic naevus syndrome

In this uncommon condition, patients have multiple large 'moles' which have a characteristic histology and a distressing propensity for malignant degeneration, particularly after prolonged exposure to strong sunshine. In these patients malignant melanoma is also more likely to develop in skin which has previously appeared normal, and this accounts for the alternative name of 'the expanded and activated melanocyte syndrome'. In some cases there is a strong

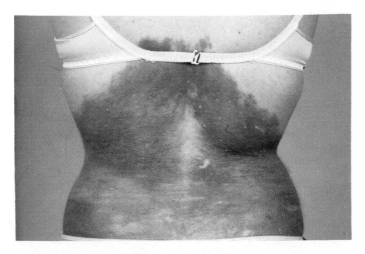

Fig. 9.9 *Tierfell* ('animal skin') melanocytic naevus

family history of malignant melanoma, and such patients obviously deserve to have frequent check-ups. They should also take care to avoid too much exposure to sunshine.

Halo naevus

Sometimes the skin around a small pigmented 'mole' becomes de-pigmented, and the 'mole' becomes paler (Fig. 9.10). Such patients have antibodies to the melanocytes, and patients with malignant melanoma sometimes develop the same antibodies. Histologically halo naevi do not show malignant changes, and their prognosis is good, but such patients have an increased risk of developing vitiligo.

Blue naevus

This is a blue-black lesion due to a collection of abnormal melan-ocytes in the deep dermis. A 'Mongolian spot' is a similar lesion over the lumbo-sacral area which is very common in infants of West Indian origin.

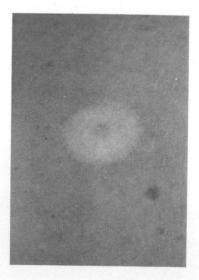

Fig. 9.10 Halo naevus

Juvenile melanoma (Spitz naevus)

This is a benign tumour of melanocytes which causes a reddish-brown nodule in children. The histology may resemble that of malignant melanoma, but the prognosis is excellent, and mutilating operations should not be performed.

2. Vascular naevi

These commonly occur at birth or shortly afterwards. There are several types, which differ in appearance and prognosis, but there is no exact clinico-histological correlation, and mixed forms are common.

a. *Telangiectatic naevi (capillary naevi).*

(i) *Salmon-patch*: A pink patch due to dilated vessels is present in about 50 per cent of newborn infants. The eyelid is a common site, and these patches fade rapidly, but those on the nape of the neck often persist.

(ii) *Port-wine stain*: This is a macular red or purple area which usually affects one side of the face. The condition persists throughout life, and can be very disfiguring. Treatment with an argon laser beam may be helpful, though the method is slow and tedious. The beam passes through the clear epidermis with little absorption and minimal damage, and is then absorbed by the abnormal dermal capillaries, causing thermal damage and thrombosis. The best results are obtained in adults rather than children, and particularly those with purple lesions. If laser therapy is not available, an expert on cosmetic camouflage should be consulted.

Occasionally a port-wine stain of the trigeminal area is associated with an underlying cerebro-vascular defect (encephalotrigeminal angiomatosis, Sturge-Weber syndrome). This may cause epilepsy or hemiparesis.

b. *Angiomatous naevi (cavernous naevi).*

A 'strawberry' mark is a small bright-red papule which develops at or soon after birth and increases in size for a few years. It then gradually involutes to leave a better end-result than can be achieved by surgery.

Rarely the angioma may be very extensive and the abnormal vessels may sequester platelets, thus causing thrombocytopenia and haemorrhage. In this situation, a short course of prednisone may be life-saving.

3. Naevus sebaceus ('organoid' naevus)

This uncommon naevus of sebaceous glands is often associated with abnormalities of the epidermis and sweat glands. It usually occurs on the scalp as a yellowish warty plaque devoid of hair, and it may undergo malignant degeneration in later life.

4. Connective tissue naevus

This is an overgrowth of dermal connective tissue which produces a soft, yellowish or skin-coloured oval plaque with an irregular surface. It usually involves the lumbosacral area, and it is often present in patients with tuberous sclerosis.

5. Epidermal naevus (Verrucous naevus)

This is a rare naevus due to epidermal hypertrophy, which usually produces a brown warty linear lesion along the length of a limb.

Many other naevi occur, but they are relatively rare, and of little clinical significance, apart from some inherited diseases in which the skin signs act as a pointer to the systemic defect:

Neurofibromatosis (von Recklinghausen's disease)

This dominantly inherited condition is characterized by multiple cafe-au-lait patches of pigmentation and multiple cutaneous neurofibromata derived from the Schwann cells of peripheral nerves (Fig. 9.11). The skin tumours are soft and dome-shaped or pedunculated. Occasionally there is a diffuse elongated fibroma along a nerve (plexiform neuroma) which may be associated with hypertrophy of the subcutaneous tissue and skin, with pendulous wrinkled folds.

The systemic features, which vary in severity, may include mental deficiency, spinal deformity, neurological lesions such as acoustic neuroma or cerebral glioma, and various endocrine diseases e.g., phaeochromocytoma.

Tuberous sclerosis (epiloia, Bourneville's disease)

The classical features of this syndrome are mental deficiency, epilepsy and cutaneous angio-fibromata which produce pink papules around the naso-labial folds. Other characteristic skin lesions are

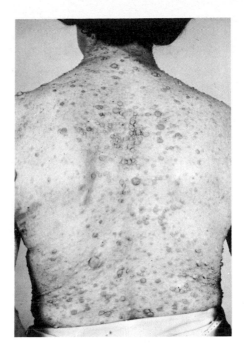

Fig. 9.11 Neurofibromatosis with multiple Schwannomas

the *shagreen patch* (a connective tissue naevus, p. 112), firm *fibromata* emerging from the nail folds, and elliptical *white macules* on the trunk which are best seen under Wood's light.

Many bizarre systemic manifestations have been reported, including ocular abnormalities, rhabdomyosarcoma and renal tumours.

10

Viral skin infections

Many systemic viral infections such as rubeola (measles), rubella
(German measles) and varicella (chicken pox) cause a characteristic
rash (the exanthem), but the following account deals mainly with
viruses which primarily invade the skin. The diagnosis in these
cases can be confirmed where necessary by sending a skin specimen
(fluid, scrapings or biopsy) to the laboratory, or in some cases, by
taking serial blood tests to detect rising antiviral antibody titres.
Serological proof of the viral aetiology may then turn up weeks
later, like some plodding detective long after the case has been
solved.

The host response is important in determining the severity of
viral infections, and the use of cytotoxic (immunosuppressive)
drugs may cause viral skin lesions to become widely disseminated.

Verruca (Wart)

Most people develop one or more viral warts at some time, and they
are especially common on the hands and feet of children. In most
patients they are a trivial self-limiting complaint, but in a few cases
they proliferate mightily and can be very difficult to eradicate.

There are at least 15 types of human papilloma virus which can
induce benign warty tumours of the skin or mucosa (genital, buccal
or laryngeal). All these viruses are identical on electron microscopy,
but they possess different antigens, and are now classified according
to their DNA base sequences. The different viruses are preferentially associated with warts of different morphology, and the various
types may need different treatments (Fig. 10.1).

1. Common warts These are firm papules with a rough hyperkeratotic surface. They may occur singly or coalesce into large
masses. The back of the hands are usually affected, and they often
cluster around the nails. They are not usually painful and most will
resolve spontaneously within two years.

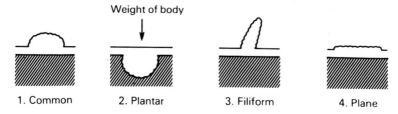

Fig. 10.1 Types of verruca

Treatment

Views on the treatment of common warts vary. Some dermatologists advise no treatment, but those afflicted tend not to share this disdain. Others rely on 'wart charms' which have a long history of successes, and some doctors successfully 'buy' the warts from small children for a few pence. One professor of dermatology claims to solve the wart problem by burying the referring doctor at the crossroads with a holly stake through his heart.

Many patients find their warts disappear with the regular application of a proprietary wart paint containing keratolytics such as salicylic and lactic acids. Unresponsive cases will usually clear by freezing them for 30–60 sec with carbon dioxide snow or liquid nitrogen, but the application may have to be repeated several times at three-weekly intervals. The treatment is painful, and over-enthusiastic freezing can produce blisters and even scars. A supply of sweets should be kept for children to transform tears to smiles. In really stubborn cases cauterization using the electric 'Hyfrecator' under local anaesthesia may be needed, and every dermatologist sees occasional patients in whom the warts would recur in the stump even if the hand was amputated. These patients probably have a defect in immune response to the wart virus, since antibody titres normally rise as the warts clear. Intralesional injection of bleomycin solution is sometimes helpful in these very stubborn cases.

2. *Plantar warts* These occur on the sole, and the body weight causes them to grow inwards rather than outwards. They are often painful on walking. They may resemble callosities (simple hyperkeratosis) but gentle paring with a scalpel will reveal a well-defined margin, often with fine bleeding points. Sometimes there are multiple shallow confluent lesions over a wide area of the sole and these are called *mosaic warts*.

Treatment
Patients usually demand treatment either because the foot is painful or because they are being excluded from the local swimming-bath. The application of a 20 per cent salicylic acid plaster to the wart surface for four days softens the keratin and allows it to be pared away. The plaster should be held in place by strapping of the stretch-fabric type. If repeated conscientiously this is usually eventually successful, but many patients fail to perform the vigorous paring which is essential. Freezing, curettage and superficial electrocautery may also be used. Heroic surgery is to be avoided as the ensuing scar may be more painful than the original wart.

Mosaic warts are often resistant to treatment, but formalin 'soaks' or 20 per cent formalin in an ointment base may be effective.

3. *Filiform warts* These are small filamentous warts, often on the face. They are easily dealt with by curettage or cauterization.

4. *Plane warts* These small flat-topped warts are often multiple and may be a cosmetic nuisance. 2 per cent salicylic acid ointment is usually effective.

5. *Condyloma acuminata* (genital warts) The responsible virus resembles the common wart virus but is antigenically distinct. The clinical appearance is also distinctive, with soft pink fleshy excrescences around the anus, the perianal area or the mucosa of the vulva or penis. Since the condition is contagious it is classed as a venereal disease, and some experts advise tests for gonorrhoea and syphilis in such patients. This precaution also helps to exclude the possibility of *condyloma lata* (p. 133) the broad flat-topped pink papules of which could be mistaken for condyloma acuminata.

Treatment
Podophyllin (15 to 25 per cent) in tincture of benzoin or in industrial methylated spirit should be painted on to the condylomata at weekly intervals. This cytotoxic drug is highly irritant to the surrounding normal skin, which should be protected by the prior application of Vaseline. The patient should also be warned to bathe the area after 8 hr, or painful chemical burns may ensure. Pregnancy causes genital warts to enlarge, but podophyllin should not be used during pregnancy as it is absorbed and may damage the fetus. In pregnancy electro-cautery of the warts is required.

Human papillomaviruses (HPV) and carcinoma

Although viral warts of the skin are almost invariably benign, cer tain types of HPV can occasionally play a role in inducing squamous carcinoma, particularly on the mucosal surfaces, and two similar viruses in animals (polyoma and simian viruses) are known to be highly oncogenic.

It is thought that genital warts can predispose to squamous carcinoma, since about 15 per cent of penile cancers arise at the site of genital warts. Renal transplant patients also have a high incidence of warts and skin cancer, and it has been suggested that both the immunosuppression and the viral infection may predispose to the carcinoma. There is also a rare condition called *epidermodysplasia verruciformis* which is characterized by generalized flat warts due to life-long HPV infection, and about 30 per cent of these patients develop skin cancer in middle life.

Herpes simplex

This common infection seems to be on everyone's lips these days. It is due to herpesvirus hominis, of which there are two distinct types (HSV-1 and HSV-2). HSV-1 commonly affects the lips and mouth. It can also cause keratitis and corneal ulceration, and rarely it causes encephalitis. HSV-2 commonly causes genital or anal lesions, but around 20 per cent of genital herpes is due to HSV-1, presumably due to oral sex. Both HSV-1 and HSV-2 can affect the skin.

Clinical features

1. *Primary herpes simplex* usually develops before the age of five, the infection being contracted from the mother. The infection may be subclinical, or there may be painful ulcers of the mouth and tongue with red swollen gums, malaise and pyrexia. In severe cases the infant will not drink, and iv infusions may be required until the condition spontaneously subsides in about 10 days.

2. *Recurrent herpes* The 'cold sore' (herpes labialis) which occurs on the lips is characterized by irritable or tingling grouped vesicles on a red base, which crust over and subside in about 7–14 days. Such lesions tend to recur every few months, and precipitating causes include pyrexia, menstruation and exposure to UVR. The virus (HSV-1) probably remains in a latent phase in the trigeminal root ganglion, and sends a constant stream of virus particles down the nerve to the skin. Normally the particles are inactivated, but prostaglandins (which are liberated by UVR) and possibly other chemical mediators enable the virus to replicate and produce clin-

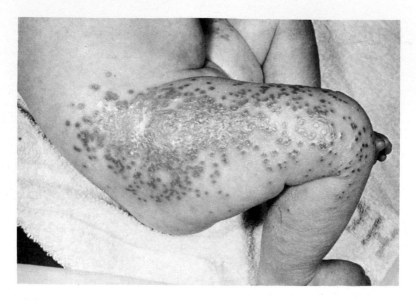

Fig. 10.2 Eczema herpeticum (Kaposi's varicelliform eruption)

ical lesions. Herpes simplex can also involve the skin in other areas, and recurrent attacks can cause scarring.

Erythema multiforme is a characteristic immunological reaction which may develop about 10 days after an overt infection with herpes simplex (p. 201).

3. Herpetic whitlow. This is an exquisitely painful condition in which the virus becomes inoculated into the skin around the nail-fold. It is prone to develop in dentists and nurses who put their ungloved fingers into many mouths.

4. Kaposi's varicelliform eruption ('eczema herpeticum') This somewhat confusing term refers to a widespread dissemination of herpes simplex lesions which resemble the lesions of varicella. It classically develops in subjects with active atopic eczema, presumably because of their relative immuno-incompetence (p. 183), but it may also occur in subjects who are immunosuppressed by drugs or other diseases. The patients are often very ill, with fever, malaise, lymphadenopathy and a widespread vesicular rash which becomes pustular and then crusts over.

A clinically indistinguishable condition can develop in patients with atopic eczema who are vaccinated against small-pox with the vaccinia virus.

5. *Genital herpes* This venereal disease mainly affects the penis, vulva and cervix, but perianal and rectal lesions are not uncommon in homosexual men. There may also be regional lymphadenopathy, malaise, fever, dysuria and frequency of micturition. More rarely, meningitis or lumbosacral radiculitis may lead to constipation or retention of urine. All patients should have routine syphilis serology, and a search for other venereal diseases.

The folklore of the media has convinced many patients that herpes is a lifelong affliction which is painful, incurable, highly contagious, and ruinous to the sex life. Females have the added benefit of death and deformity of their babies, with cervical cancer to follow later. Like many fairy-stories, this cannot be completely denied, and it may be true that the main difference between true love and herpes is that herpes lasts longer, but patients can be reassured that: (1) In many people the condition runs a benign course and the attacks eventually stop altogether. (2) Most patients are not infectious when there are no lesions present. (3) Neonatal herpes is rare, but for mothers shedding virus near to term, Caesarean section can be performed. (4). Regular cervical smears can greatly diminish the worry of cervical cancer. Genital herpes certainly provides an effective excuse for those who want to say 'No', but as a fairy story, it cannot compete with AIDS.

Treatment of herpes simplex

Many herpetic lesions are mild and transient and need no treatment. For recurrent 'cold sores' the application of a topical antiseptic or even ether may accelerate resolution by preventing secondary infection. The specific anti-viral agent 5-iodo-deoxyuridine (5 IDU) which blocks viral replication may be used for more severe lesions which are causing scarring or recurrent pain. It is usually used as a 5–20 per cent solution in dimethysulphoxide (DMSO). This is a vehicle which greatly enhances penetration through the horny layer, which is normally an effective barrier. This must be applied as soon as possible after the lesion appears, and should be repeated at four hourly intervals for several days. This will hasten resolution and help to prevent recurrence. Ophthalmic herpes ('dendritic ulcers') can be treated with aqueous IDU solution.

Acyclovir is a new drug which blocks viral replication without affecting normal cell division. It is activated only by an enzyme (thymidine kinase) produced by the virus, so that the virus in effect activates the agent which destroys it, and cellular DNA synthesis is not affected. The drug is effective orally and topically against *herpesvirus hominis* and *varicella* virus. Its value for routine use is still debatable, though if used early in the attacks it seems to abort the sores and reduce the healing-time.

Kaposi's varicelliform eruption poses a special problem, and it can sometimes be fatal. No adequately controlled trials have been reported, but pooled gamma globulin injections and systemic infusion of adenine arabinoside (Ara–A) may be beneficial.

Herpes zoster ('Shingles')

This painful blistering rash (confined to one or more dermatomes) is caused by the varicella virus. It is thought that following childhood infection with chicken-pox the virus remains dormant for many years in a dorsal root ganglion until some stimulus such as decreased host immunity induces spread of virus to the corresponding dermatome. No age is immune, but it is most common in the middle-aged and elderly. Small children may develop chickenpox after exposure to a patient with 'shingles'.

The individual lesions resemble herpes simplex, with multiple uniform vesicles on a red base (Fig. 10.3). The vesicles rapidly rupture and form crusted lesions which slowly heal in about two weeks. Secondary bacterial infection with pustule formation is common, and scarring may result. The typical rash is easily recognized by its unilateral band-like distribution with a sharp 'cut-off' in the midline. The diagnosis is easily missed even by experienced physicians in less commonly affected areas such as the S4 dermatome (perianal) particularly if, as often happens, there are one or two isolated varicella lesions elsewhere on the body. Severe pain may precede the appearance of the rash by 24–48 hours and most general practitioners have at some time diagnosed pleurisy or 'pulled muscle' in a patient who returns two days later to say that his wife has diagnosed 'shingles'. The pain may persist for months or even years after the rash has cleared, especially in the elderly, and this *postherpetic neuralgia* can be so distressing as to produce suicidal depression.

Ophthalmic zoster Any of the three divisions of the trigeminal nerve (ophthalmic, maxillary or mandibular) may be involved in herpes zoster, and if the naso-ciliary branch of the ophthalmic division is affected serious ocular complications may ensue. These include conjunctivitis, scleritis, keratitis, iritis and glaucoma. Ex-

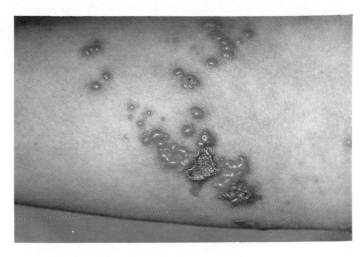

Fig. 10.3 Herpes zoster at an early stage

pert advice on management is essential and treatment may include antibiotics, analgesics, topical steroid eyedrops and IDU.

The inflammatory process may spread into the motor root, and some degree of residual ocular or facial palsy is common.

Geniculate zoster (Ramsay-Hunt syndrome) This rarity produces a painful ear, deafness, facial palsy and taste loss due to involvement of the geniculate ganglion.

Disseminated zoster ('generalized varicella') Patients with malignancy or those who have received immunosuppressive drugs are more likely to develop herpes zoster, and in such patients the eruption may become generalized. The lesions are often necrotic and haemorrhagic, and involvement of the lungs and meninges may cause death.

Treatment of herpes zoster

The application of 40 per cent 5-IDU in DMSO will hasten resolution but the treatment is expensive, and continued application of DMSO to large areas of skin may produce side-effects such as ulceration. Acyclovir may also be helpful, and for disseminated zoster it should be given intravenously. Secondary bacterial infection should be prevented with a topical antiseptic such as dibromopropamidine cream and analgesics should be given as necessary. The risk of the development of post-herpetic neuralgia is reduced if prednisone 40 mg daily is given in the first few days of the rash.

Post-herpetic neuralgia is intractable, but remedies which are worth trying include oral carbamazepine ('Tegretol'), local anaesthetic injection, local vibrators and surgical nerve root division.

Molluscum contagiosum

This pox virus produces a crop of firm pink pearly papules, some of which have a distinctive central depression (Fig. 10.4). They occur on the trunk or face and may need treatment for cosmetic reasons. They eventually resolve spontaneously, but any destructive procedure such as the application of liquid nitrogen or phenol will hasten their demise.

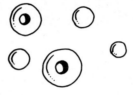

Fig. 10.4 Central umbilication of molluscum contagiosum

The histology of these lesions gives pleasure to pathologists, since the central cells of the lesion become distended with masses of pink-staining material to produce unforgettable 'molluscum bodies'.

Hand, foot and mouth disease

This disease is produced by only a few strains of the Coxsackie virus. The rash consists of a few isolated vesicles often in a linear arrangement on the palms and soles, with shallow mouth ulcers which are often painful (Fig. 10.5). Young children are the usual victims, and the condition clears in 10 days. It is important to realize that this disease is not related to foot and mouth disease in cattle, and it is therefore not necessary to shoot patients and bury them in a pit of quick-lime.

Orf

Orf is primarily a disease of sheep, in which it produces pustules around the muzzle. It can be transmitted to humans in whom it produces a single large purple painful swelling (Fig. 10.6). The typical patient has bottle-fed infected lambs, develops a single lesion

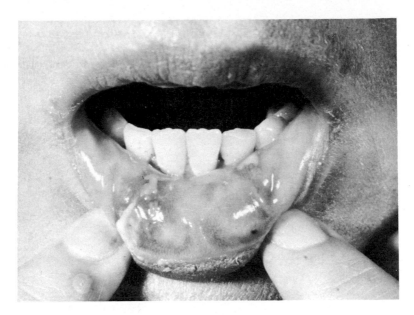

Fig. 10.5 Hand, foot and mouth disease. Note the blister on the finger

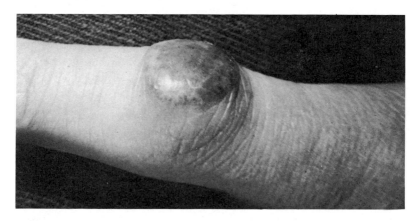

Fig. 10.6 Orf on the finger

on the finger and knows the diagnosis but requires reassurance. Uninitiated doctors usually misdiagnose the lesion as anthrax. The diagnosis can be confirmed by electron microscopy of the vesicle fluid. Spontaneous healing occurs in about three weeks, but *erythema multiforme* (p. 201) is a notoriously common complication.

Cowpox and milkers' nodules

Electrocution by the milking machine has now largely replaced these traditional hazards of the dairymaid. Cowpox produces scattered pustules with fever, malaise and lymphadenopathy, and milkers' nodules are brownish-purple lumps which develop on the fingers.

Pityriasis rosea

The word 'pityriasis', derived from the Greek for bran husks, is applied to many dermatoses with delicate pellucid scales — pityriasis rosea, pityriasis alba (p. 31), pityriasis versicolor (p. 141), pityriasis capitis (p. 51), etc.

Pityriasis rosea is a common, self-limiting, distinctive eruption of young adults. It is presumed to be due to a virus, but no organism has been regularly isolated. The first sign is the appearance of an oval red scaly patch, usually situated on the trunk, some 2 to 5 cm in diameter. This *herald patch* is followed after an interval of 5 to 15 days by a generalized eruption of smaller discrete patches, mainly over the trunk, but spreading on to the upper arms and thighs. Each patch is yellowish-pink with a collarette of fine scales, and they are characteristically distributed in lines parallel to the ribs (Fig. 10.7).

There may be mild pruritus, and occasional malaise and lymphadenopathy. The rash fades away after about six weeks, and although no treatment is needed beyond antipruritics and reassurance, it tends to clear more quickly with UV irradiation.

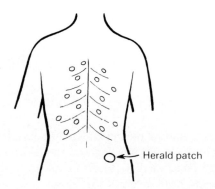

Fig. 10.7 'Christmas-tree' distribution of pityriasis rosea

The typical rash is easy to diagnose, but many atypical cases occur and in these patients secondary syphilis must be excluded by a WR test. Secondary syphilis often looks like pityriasis rosea. It too affects young adults, and it causes malaise and lymphadenopathy. The doctor who labels this as pityriasis rosea will congratulate himself when the rash clears spontaneously, but he may blush at his error when the patient returns some years later with tertiary syphilis (but more likely he will misdiagnose this too, and congratulate himself again).

11

Bacterial infections

THE FLORA AND FAUNA OF THE SKIN

The skin varies considerably from one part of the body to another, and the varying terrains and micro-climates of the skin surface have been fancifully but memorably compared to the different regions of the earth, each with its characteristic flora and fauna. Thus the scalp is a thick, dark wood which shades and protects the numerous bacteria and yeasts on its surface, the forehead is a sun-baked plain which yet supports a heavy growth of anaerobes in the depths of the follicles, the nail plate is a barren desert which resists bacterial colonization, and the sweaty warm axilla is a tropical rain forest which teems with life.

Organisms which are commonly found on normal skin as commensals include the Gram-negative *Staphylococcus albus*, various *diphtheroids*, yeasts such as *Pityrosporum ovale*, and the mite, *Demodex folliculorum*. Some of these commensals are found in increased numbers in dermatoses such as seborrhoeic dermatitis, acne vulgaris and rosacea but their role in pathogenesis is debatable, since Koch's postulates have not been fulfilled and the diseases might themselves encourage secondary proliferation of the organisms.

Other organisms such as Staphylococcus aureus, β-haemolytic Streptococci and Proteus are usually pathogens, but when they are isolated from a damaged skin surface such as a leg ulcer it can be difficult to assess whether they are causing inflammation or are merely passive contaminants.

Finally, there are organisms such as Treponema pallidum and Mycobacterium tuberculosis which are always of diagnostic importance when they are isolated from the skin.

DISEASES DUE TO STAPHYLOCOCCI

1. Furuncle and carbuncle

A furuncle ('boil') is a deep abscess of a hair follicle due to Staphylococcus aureus. It begins as a red, tender papule which rapidly develops into a large painful *pustule*, which 'points' and discharges a greenish-yellow core. 'Boils' are common in young men, and the back of the neck, axillae and buttocks are the usual sites. Precipitating factors may include poor hygiene, stress and diabetes mellitus, but 'boils' often recur at intervals for no apparent reason. Such patients often carry the Staphylococci in the nose, axillae and groins between attacks, and such 'carriers' can be a menace in an operating theatre.

A *carbuncle* is a confluent mass of 'boils' which usually indicates an underlying debility.

Treatment

A single 'boil' should be treated initially with frequent local heat, and with a magnesium sulphate paste dressing after it has burst. 'Carriers' should be treated with antiseptic nasal cream (e.g., Naseptin) and daily chlorhexidine baths, and a prolonged course of flucloxacillin may help to prevent recurrences.

A carbuncle is a serious illness which, if neglected, can lead to Staphylococcal septicaemia. Systemic flucloxacillin is required, with incision of the purulent abscesses.

2. Impetigo

Impetigo is a superficial, rapidly spreading skin infection due to Staphylococcus aureus, often with β-haemolytic streptococci in addition. An established case is easily recognized by the dirty-looking crusted appearance of the lesion, but in the early stages clear bullae may develop in apparently normal skin, especially in young children. The bulla develops from the action of an epidermolytic toxin on the granular layer. If the toxin becomes widely disseminated in the bloodstream, it produces generalized toxic epidermal necrolysis (p. 128). Impetigo is very contagious especially in children, and it becomes epidemic in over-crowded households, particularly if towels are shared. Lice, scabies and eczema are common predisposing conditions and sometimes all four disease occur in the same patient. In some areas (e.g., the West Indies) glomerulonephritis commonly complicates Streptococcal impetigo, but this is rare in Britain.

Treatment

An antibiotic cream such as chlortetracycline should be applied to the lesions several times daily, and if the condition is extensive or the home conditions are poor, oral penicillin (unless the organism is resistant) should also be given.

3. Infantile toxic epidermal necrolysis ('Scalded skin' syndrome)

Pathogenic Staphylococci of specific phage types (e.g., 71) liberate exotoxins which can be shown to produce widespread erythema and sloughing of the epidermis in baby mice but have no effect in adult mice. Human infants infected with these strains develop a similar widespread epidermal necrolysis which mimics clinically the effect of boiling water on the skin. Though rare, it is important that this life-threatening condition is recognized, since it responds well to appropriate antibiotic therapy.

4. Sycosis barbae

This is a chronic deep-seated folliculitis of the beard area in men. Staphylococci can sometimes be isolated, but often the lesions are sterile, and the response to antibiotics may be poor. Long term oral tetracyclines and topical antiseptics are sometimes useful, but some cases grumble on for years.

DISEASES DUE TO STREPTOCOCCI

Erysipelas

This is a superficial infection with Streptococcus pyogenes, which produces a sharply marginated, red, tender, oedematous area which steadily spreads. There may be red streaks of lymphangitis, with regional lymphadenopathy, and the patient often feels ill and feverish. The organism usually gains entry to the skin through an ulcer or crack in the epidermis (e.g., caused by tinea pedis). Impairment of the lymphatic drainage predisposes to erysipelas. *Cellulitis* is a deeper Streptococcal infection involving the subcutaneous tissues, but the two conditions overlap.

Treatment

Intramuscular penicillin is the treatment of choice, since Streptococci are very rarely resistant. Erysipelas may be recurrent, in which case long-term penicillin may be used prophylactically.

DISEASES DUE TO DIPHTHEROIDS

1. Acne vulgaris

There is some evidence that *Propionibacterium acnes* plays a central role in this disease (see p. 59), even though it is a commensal organism in many adults.

2. Erythrasma

Erythrasma is characterized by patches of erythema and slight scaling in the axillae and groins, which are often mistaken for tinea. The causative organisms are diphtheroids which produce porphyrins, so that the lesions fluoresce coral-pink under Woods's light. The condition responds to oral erythromycin or topical miconazole cream.

3. Trichomycosis axillaris

Despite its name, this condition is not due to fungus intection, but is merely an orange discoloration of the axillary hairs due to overgrowth of diphtheroids on the hair shafts.

4. Pitted keratolysis

This is an unusual condition in which diphtheroid overgrowth on the soles of sweaty feet produces a striking 'geographical' pattern of shallow keratinolysis. It responds well to formalin soaks.

DISEASES DUE TO MYCOBACTERIA

1. Cutaneous tuberculosis

This is becoming increasingly rare with the decline in systemic TB.

(i) *Lupus vulgaris* is a slowly progressive, post-primary infection which occurs in subjects with a relatively high degree of immunity to the M. tuberculosis bacillus. The organisms are therefore sparse in the skin but the Mantoux reaction is strongly positive. The characteristic lesion is a rather translucent reddish-brown plaque (Fig. 11.1), often on the face, which enlarges over the years, causing considerable scarring and destruction of underlying tissue such as nasal cartilage. The response to isoniazid is good, and resistance is very rare.

(ii) *'Warty tuberculosis'* is an indolent verrucous plaque due to inoculation of the bacilli into the skin of a previously-infected patient. It classically occurs on the hands of pathologists and butchers.

(iii) *Papulonecrotic tuberculid* is an eruption of necrotic papules which usually occur in crops on the extremities of young adults. It is an immunological response to tuberculosis elsewhere in the body, and although bacilli are not found in the skin, the condition clears with anti-tuberculous therapy.

Many other forms occur, but are now very rare in Britain.

2. Leprosy (Hansen's disease)

Though leprosy (due to Mycobacterium leprae) is not endemic in Britain it is occasionally seen in immigrants from India, Africa and Asia. There are several clinical types, which are determined by the immunological status of the host, as follows:

Tuberculoid	Borderline	Lepromatous
TT←→BT←→BB←→BL←→LL		
(marked cell-mediated immunity to M. leprae)		(poor cell-mediated immunity to M. leprae)

Tuberculoid leprosy usually presents as a single circumscribed anaesthetic hypopigmented macule with decreased sweat production and loss of hair in the affected area. The superficial nerves may be thickened and readily palpable. Skin smears for acid-fast bacilli are negative, but the lepromin skin test shows a strong Type 4 hypersensitivity reaction.

Lepromatous leprosy usually presents with multiple, reddish shiny lesions which are not anaesthetic. There is often a severe peripheral neuropathy and considerable tissue damage. Loss of the eyebrows is a characteristic sign. There are many bacilli in the skin smears, but the lepromin test is negative.

Borderline leprosy shows features of both the above types, and varies widely in its manifestations.

Indeterminate leprosy is an uncommon transitory phase (which

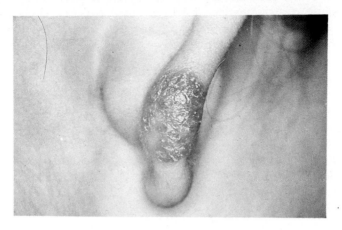

Fig. 11.1 Lupus vulgaris

may last for months) in which the immunological status has not yet been determined.

Leprosy is probably transmitted by droplets from the upper respiratory tract of patients with lepromatous leprosy, and the incubation period is several years.

Treatment

The treatment of leprosy demands considerable expertise as severe reactions to therapy can occur. Most cases require dapsone therapy, which is continued for at least five years. Resistance to dapsone has recently become a problem in some countries, and other drugs such as rifampicin or ethionamide may be required. Development of a vaccine has been hampered by the fact that the organism grows only in cool tissues and cannot be cultured *in vitro*. Experimental transmission in animals is difficult but the nine-banded armadillo, which has an unusually low body temperature, has recently been successfully used as a host.

3. Swimming pool granuloma (Fish-tank granuloma)

The so-called '*atypical Mycobacteria*' such as M. marinum occasionally cause chronic indolent bluish nodular lesions when they are inoculated into human skin. Patients often recall scrambling from a poorly chlorinated pool or cutting themselves while cleaning a tank which has contained sick fish. The diagnosis is easily missed by routine bacteriological testing, since the organisms grow only at low temperatures.

4. Buruli ulcer

This tropical disease produces a large ulcer with undermined edges. It usually occurs on the legs of children. It is due to M. ulcerans, and is unusual in being transmitted by spiky grass, which in swampy districts (e.g., Buruli) harbours the bacilli which are then inoculated into the bare legs of passers-by.

DISEASES DUE TO TREPONEMATA

1. Syphilis (Lues)

Infection with *Treponema pallidum* may be congenital or acquired. Since it can invade every organ, syphilis has a reputation for mimicking other diseases. The cutaneous manifestations are as follows:

(i) *Primary chancre*

This is an indurated, flat, disc-shaped inflamed lesion which on squeezing exudes serum containing numerous T. pallidum organisms. It may occur anywhere on the penis, vulva, vagina, cervix, anus or rectum and occasionally the buccal mucosa, nipple or finger may be involved. The primary chancre usually develops from 10 days to 3 weeks after infection, but the WR does not become positive for 4 to 6 weeks.

(ii) *Secondary syphilis*

This is the stage of generalized involvement, which occurs from 8 weeks to 2 years after infection. It is usually accompanied by constitutional symptoms (e.g., headache, fever, malaise), a widespread rash and lesions of the mucous membranes. The rash has a variety of appearances, and may mimic many other skin diseases, particularly pityriasis rosea, but it never blisters, it rarely itches, and it often involves the palms. The rash is sometimes a very faint pink, and can be seen only in natural light, although some patients may be covered in scaly indurated copper-coloured papules.

Condylomata lata (singular, condyloma latum) are broad, moist, pink papules which commonly occur around the ano-genital area or lips in secondary syphilis. In the mouth there may be smooth patches on the tongue, papular lesions (known as *'mucous patches'*) on the buccal mucosa, with tonsillitis and linear grey erosions called *'snail-track ulcers'* in the pharynx. These mucosal lesions are all highly infectious.

Occasional patients have alopecia (p. 47).

General examination may reveal pyrexia, generalized lymphadenopathy, mild jaundice or uveitis.

(iii) *Tertiary syphilis*

A *gumma*, now rarely seen, may develop in the skin as a single painless nodule which eventually ulcerates. On the legs the ulcer can be mistaken for a venous ulcer, but the characteristic scalloped edge and yellow 'wash-leather' slough in the base should suggest the need for biopsy and serological tests.

(iv) *Congenital syphilis*

The infection is transmitted across the placenta, and congenital syphilis is rarely seen in countries where ante-natal WR tests are performed routinely.

The cutaneous lesions may be macular, papular or bullous, and the palms are always involved. Linear fissures at the angles of the mouth leave characteristic scars called *rhagades* in later life.

Treatment of syphilis

Penicillin is the drug of choice, but treatment should be supervised by a specialist with facilities for contact tracing.

2. Non-venereal treponematoses

These include *yaws, endemic syphilis* ('bejel') and *pinta*. They usually affect children in rural parts of tropical or subtropical areas. They have similar clinical features, with skin lesions predominating. Serological tests for syphilis are positive, and they respond well to penicillin.

DISEASES DUE TO NEISSERIA

1. Gonococcal dermatitis

About 1 per cent of patients with gonorrhoea (due to *Neisseria gonorrhoeae*) develop a gonococcaemia, with fever, arthritis and scattered skin lesions, which may be either small maculo-papules, pustules, haemorrhagic papules or tender nodules. Genito-urinary manifestations may be minimal, but complement fixation blood tests for gonorrhoea are usually positive.

2. Meningococcal septicaemia

Meningococcaemia (due to *Neisseria meningitidis*) causes a feverish illness which may cause death within hours, or may produce only episodic symptoms for several weeks. The more acute forms are commonly accompanied by a widespread purpuric rash, which occurs in crops. A transient morbilliform rash may also occur. In fulminating cases there may be extensive ecchymoses.

ANTHRAX

This disease, due to *Bacillus anthracis*, is now rare in Britain. It causes a large painful, purple swelling, which is accompanied by fever, headache and malaise. Death can occur within days, but the prognosis is good if i.m. penicillin is given early. The bacilli can be identified in stained smears, and subsequently confirmed by animal inoculation. Anthrax is an occupational hazard of men handling imported animal products (bone-meal, hides, wood, etc.) but has also been reported in bongo-drum beaters.

12

Fungal infections

Fungi affect the lives of most people. They destroy a proportion of our crops, they produce antibiotics, they are used for brewing and baking and they commonly infect human beings.

The fungi responsible for human disease may be multicellular filaments, *hyphae*, which reproduce by spore formation, or unicellular *yeasts* which reproduce by budding.

Deep mycoses (fungal infections) invade living tissue and cause systemic disease (e.g., histoplasmosis, actinomycosis) but *superficial mycoses* are usually confined to the skin and mucous membranes.

SUPERFICIAL MYCOSES.

A. Dermatophyte infections

Dermatophytes are filamentous fungi which digest keratin by enzymes. They therefore attack skin, hair and nails, but they cannot invade living cells. There are many species which vary in their geographical distribution and in their predilection for different sites, but there are only three main families:

1. Microsporum
2. Trichophyton
3. Epidermophyton

The *anthropophilic* species are virtually confined to man, but the *zoophilic* species primarily affect animals and only occasionally infect humans. The host reaction to dermatophytes is very variable. The anthropophilic species tend to live in symbiosis with man, causing relatively little inflammation and pursuing a very chronic course, whereas the zoophilic species excite an intense but short-lived inflammatory reaction, often with vesicles and pustules.

1. Tinea pedis ('Athlete's foot')

This condition is commonest in adult males, particularly those who wear heavy footwear, work in a hot environment and share communal bathing facilities. It usually starts as a patch of macerated irritable skin between the 4th and 5th toes and gradually spreads to the soles and dorsum of the foot. There may be only minimal redness and scaling, or there may be an acute vesicular or pustular eruption.

2. Tinea unguium

The infection starts distally and affects one or more, but rarely all, of the nails. The nail plate becomes thickened, discoloured and friable. Brownish discoloration of the great toe-nail is commonly due to a nondermatophyte fungus whose importance scarcely merits the grandeur of its title, Scopulariopsis brevicaulis.

3. Tinea corporis

This is the typical 'ringworm' of the trunk, face or limbs, with circular scaly lesions which clear centrally and slowly spread like ripples (Fig. 12.1). Many atypical forms occur however, particularly after steroid ointments have been used. There may be little scaling and papules or pustules may develop. The condition usually affects children, and the fungus is often caught from pets or farm animals.

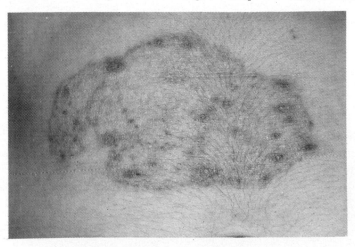

Fig. 12.1 Tinea corporis. The sharp edge is characteristic

4. *Tinea cruris*

This causes well-demarcated redness and scaling of the groins and upper thighs. It predominantly affects young men, especially athletic types who sweat and share towels. The popular term 'dhobi itch' is a misnomer. A 'dhobi' is an Indian washerwoman and soldiers used to believe the rash was due to inadequate rinsing of suds from their underpants.

5. *Tinea capitis* (*Scalp ringworm*)

The characteristic signs of this condition are circular bald patches with redness, scaling and brittle hair stumps in the patches. Some species (especially Microsporum) cause the infected hair to fluoresce green under Wood's ultra-violet light. The disease is now relatively uncommon in Britain, but before griseofulvin therapy was introduced it used to spread in epidemics through classes of schoolchildren.

Adult scalps are relatively resistant to the anthropophilic species, but 'animal ringworm' may be caught (e.g., by leaning the head on the flank of an infected cow during milking) and these zoophilic species cause a marked inflammatory reaction called a kerion (Fig. 12.2). Confluent suppurating abscesses with a tender regional lymphadenopathy are characteristic, and this may suggest a staphylococcal infection, but swabs for bacteria are usually negative.

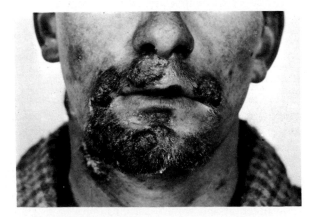

Fig. 12.2 Kerion in a farm worker

6. Tinea barbae

This refers to dermatophyte infection of the beard area.

7. 'Ide' eruption

Patients with tinea pedis occasionally develop an eczematous eruption of the hands which does not contain fungus but which clears when the tinea pedis is eradicated. This so-called 'ide' eruption is presumably an immunological reaction. Occasionally other 'ide' eruptions, e.g., follicular papules, develop transiently during treatment.

Diagnosis of dermatophyte infections

Direct microscopical examination of the infected tissue, with subsequent culture on Sabouraud's medium is advisable. Skin scrapings, nail clippings or plucked hairs should be examined after gentle heating in a drop of potassium hydroxide solution on a slide to 'clear' the keratin. The hyphae can then (with practice) be seen as parallel lines, but culture of another specimen is necessary for species identification. The specimens can conveniently be wrapped in black paper and sent to a Mycology Laboratory, by post if necessary, as the fungi remain viable for some days.

Treatment of dermatophyte infections

There are several drugs which are effective topically against dermatophytes (tolnaftate, clotrimazole and miconazole) and they are less irritant than the time-honoured Whitfield's ointment, which may provoke an eczematous reaction. Toe web infections are difficult to cure unless the patient bathes daily, dries the skin thoroughly with a rough towel, and wears cool footwear.

Griseofulvin (fine particle) 500 mg daily after a meal is specific for dermatophytes and should be used for severe or persistent infection and for tinea unguium. Finger nails may need six months' treatment, and toe nails may never completely clear even after several years' treatment.

Kerion needs vigorous therapy to prevent scarring and permanent alopecia. Griseofulvin is essential, with antibiotics for secondary bacterial infection and topical starch poultices. A short course of systemic steroids helps to suppress the inflammatory response.

B. Candidosis

Candida albicans is a yeast which is a gut commensal in most of the normal population. Under certain conditions it invades the skin or mucous membranes as a pathogen, and the following factors predispose to Candidosis:

1. Local trauma or maceration e.g., dentures, moist body folds
2. Broad-spectrum antibiotics which reduce the normal gut bacteria and allow overgrowth of Candida
3. Steroid or immunosuppressive therapy
4. Pregnancy or infancy
5. Any severe illness such as malignancy, malabsorption, TB or diabetes mellitus
6. Iron deficiency
7. Congenital immunological deficiency.

Candida albicans is better than most physicians at recognising when a person is not well.

The diagnosis of Candidosis can be confirmed if necessary by direct microscopy and culture of affected tissue (skin scraping, oral or vaginal swab or nail clipping).

Several clinical patterns occur:

1. Mucosal Candidosis ('Thrush')

Oral 'thrush' produces white patches on the buccal mucosa which can be scraped off to leave a bright red base. It occurs most commonly in babies, denture-wearers and the debilitated. Treatment with Amphotericin B Lozenges is effective if they are sucked slowly with the dentures removed.

Angular stomatitis (fissures at the corners of the lips) (Fig. 12.3) is hardly ever due to riboflavin deficiency, as examination candidates regularly suggest, but it is commonly due to Candidosis in patients with ill-fitting dentures. Other organisms such as Staphylococci and Streptococci are also often present. Iron deficiency may be present in some patients. It responds to Nystaform HC ointment, and attention to the dentures.

Vaginal 'thrush' produces a creamy discharge, with vaginal inflammation and pruritus vulvae. Pregnancy, oral contraceptives and diabetes mellitus are common predisposing factors. Treatment is with Nystatin pessaries, and it is advisable to give oral Nystatin (500 000 units b.d.) in addition in order to eradicate Candida from the bowel and prevent reinfection.

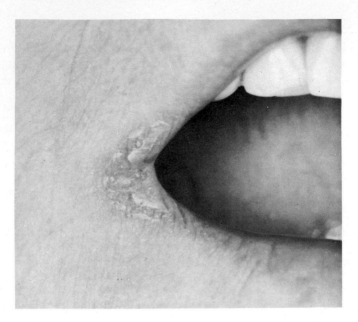

Fig. 12.3 Angular stomatitis

In the male, Candidosis can cause *balanitis* (inflammation of the foreskin) and the infection can be transmitted by sexual intercourse.

2. *Cutaneous Candidosis*

This typically involves areas of warm moist skin such as the body folds or the napkin area in infants. The rash consists of well-demarcated brick-red areas with slight peripheral scaling or vesiculation with a few outlying 'satellite' lesions (Fig. 12.4)

Nappy rash (diaper dermatitis) may be due to Candidosis, or to the irritant effect of ammonia, produced from urea by bacteria if the napkin is not changed often enough. These two possibilities can be distinguished by observing whether the depths of the skin folds are spared. Ammonia tends not to reach the depths of the folds, whereas Candida thrives there.

Nystaform HC ointment (Nystatin with Vioform and Hydrocortisone) is very effective against cutaneous Candidosis.

3. *Chronic paronychia*

This is an occupational hazard of barmaids, charladies, fish-sellers

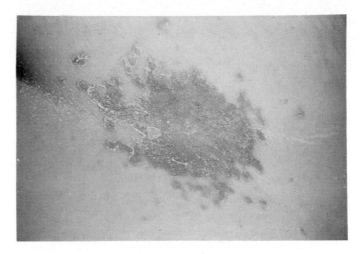

Fig. 12.4 Candidosis. Note the small satellite lesions

and others who frequently immerse their hands in water. The nail fold becomes red, swollen and tender, the cuticle is lost and pus may often be expressed from the cavity which forms beneath the nail fold

Candida albicans is the commonest infecting organism but other pathogens may occasionally be found.

Successful treatment depends on keeping the hands dry and pushing Nystatin ointment into the 'cave' of pus with a wedge-shaped orange-stick (it sounds painful but it isn't).

Occasionally the nail-plate itself may become infected with Candida, which produces a greenish-blue discoloration.

4. Chronic muco-cutaneous granulomatous Candidosis

This rare but spectacular condition affects children with a congenital immune deficiency state. Large granulomatous lesions develop on the fingers and toes, and there is often intractable oral 'thrush'. The cutaneous lesions will not heal with conventional therapy such as Nystatin, but some cases have improved following infusion of 'transfer factor' derived from lymphocytes.

C. Pityriasis versicolor

This trivial macular rash is due to a yeast called Pityrosporum orbiculare. It mainly affects young adults, and it causes a profusion of small macules on the trunk or upper arms, usually with some fine scaling. The macules may be pale brown, pink or depigmented (hence the name), and the rash usually causes no symptoms other than anxiety regarding its cause. It becomes particularly noticeable after tanning, since the affected patches remain pale.

The diagnosis can be confirmed by microscopic examination of skin scrapings. The daily application of selenium sulphide solution (Selsun shampoo) or 10 per cent sodium thiosulphate solution will eradicate the yeast. Treatment must be continued for six weeks, but the depigmented areas return to normal more slowly, and the infection often recurs a few months later.

13

Dermatoses due to parasites, insects, etc

A. WORMS AND PROTOZOA

PARASITIC WORMS

1. Oxyuriasis (threadworm, pinworm)

The commonest human worm is *Enterobius vermicularis*. Its distribution is world-wide and often whole families or communities are infested. It lives in the gut, but during sleep, the female worm, which is only about 1 cm long, emerges from the anus and wriggles over the perianal skin depositing eggs. The resultant itching causes restlessness and scratching, and re-infection occurs when the eggs are transferred to the mouth via the nails. The diagnosis can be confirmed by applying Scotch tape to the perineum, when the ova which adhere to it can be identified microscopically.

Treatment

Piperazine citrate (Antepar) or adipate (Entacyl) is given as an eight day course. Alternatively viprinium (Vanquin) may be given as a single dose, repeated after two weeks, but this drug colours the stools red and may cause nausea.

2. Toxocariasis

This is an infestation with the larvae of the common roundworm of dogs (Toxocara canis) or cats (Toxocara catis). Skin tests show that about 2 per cent of the British population becomes infested during early childhood, probably as a result of playing in soil contaminated with animal excreta. The ova are ingested and the resultant larvae migrate from the gut to most parts of the body and die. Most human infestations are asymptomatic, but occasionally

143

generalized pruritus and urticaria with eosinophilia may occur. The disease may rarely cause cough, myalgia, epilepsy, blindness, etc.

The following worms and protozoa are not endemic in Britain. Larger texts must be consulted if details of diagnostic tests and treatment are required.

3. Filariasis (Tropical elephantiasis)

Infestation with the filarial worms *Wuchereria bancrofti* and *Brugia malayi* is common throughout the tropics. The disease is transmitted by mosquitoes which inject the larvae into the blood. These migrate and mature, and the adult worms live in the lymphatics, whence the fertilized females discharge microfilariae, chiefly at night, into the blood. After a prolonged incubation period affected patients develop lymphangitis and recurrent fever, and eventually the defective lymphatic drainage causes *elephantiasis* (massive, non-pitting oedema and fibrosis of the skin) of the legs and scrotum.

4. Onchocerciasis (Blinding filariasis)

This infestation with the filarial worm *Onchocerea volvulus* occurs most commonly in tropical Africa and the disease vectors are small flies. The affected patients develop pruritus, a papular rash with dermal nodules, and, in severe cases, blindness.

5. Dracunculosis (Guinea worm)

Humans in Asia and Africa may acquire this disease by drinking water containing water-fleas infested with larvae of the worm *Dranunculus medinensis*. The larvae migrate through the intestinal wall and eventually reach the skin of the lower leg. The adult female worm then causes a red papule to develop, which blisters over 24 hours, and under the stimulus of contact with water, a milky fluid is discharged which contains enormous quantities of larvae. There is often a constitutional upset, with malaise, fever and urticaria.

6. Larva migrans (Creeping eruption)

This is a distinctive eruption which is due to the larvae of various worms such as *Ankylostoma braziliense* and *Strongyloides stercoralis*. The larvae penetrate human skin and migrate beneath the surface, leaving an itchy, red, raised line. This may extend by several cm daily to produce a bizarre, convoluted track.

PROTOZOA

1. Leishmaniasis

Flagellate protozoa of the *Leishmania* species are widely distributed in hot climates.

Cutaneous Leishmaniasis is endemic around the Mediterranean coast, and is occasionally imported to Britain by unlucky holiday-makers. The disease is transmitted by sandflies and the incubation period may be several months. Several clinical forms occur, but often a large reddish-brown papule, nodule or ulcer develops on the face.

Visceral Leishmaniasis (kala-azar) affects children in the tropics and causes fever, emaciation, hepato-splenomegaly, anaemia and patchy hyperpigmentation.

2. Amoebiasis

Cutaneous amoebiasis occurs in countries such as Mexico where *Entamoeba histolytica* is common. The condition develops either by extension from amoebic dysentry or by direct inoculation into the skin. The ulcerating skin lesions spread rapidly and cause death if untreated.

B. ARTHROPODS

Included in the phylum Arthropoda are the Hexapoda (true insects) and the Arachnida (mites, ticks, spiders and scorpions) and hundreds of species in these two classes can cause skin disease by one or more of the following mechanisms:

1. Mechanical trauma from bites or stings (e.g., horse-flies)
2. Injection of toxins (e.g., bees)
3. Hypersensitization to a substance which comes in contact with, or is injected into, the skin. Various types of immune responses (e.g., I, III or IV) may be involved (p. 207).
4. Invasion of the skin by the arthropod (e.g., maggots).
5. Transmission of another disease by the arthropod (e.g., leishmaniasis by sand-flies).
6. Secondary bacterial invasion (e.g., impetigo from lice).

INSECTS

'Papular urticaria' ('heat bumps')

This confusing term refers to a chronic or recurrent eruption of intensely itchy urticated papules which are often grouped, and tend to be seasonal. The lesions develop in crops, each lasting for about 4 to 14 days, and they tend to leave a pigmented scar. The new papules often have a central haemorrhagic punctum.

This clinical picture is probably always due to insect bites. The culprit often cannot be identified but fleas and bed-bugs are common causes. Increased host sensitivity is probably important, since only one member of the family may be affected. The condition gradually clears, possibly due to desensitization following repeated bites, because children often improve just as a younger sibling begins to develop the disease.

Insect bites from gnats and midges etc. may produce other clinical patterns e.g., one or more large bullae (up to 5 cm) may develop suddenly on the lower leg (Fig. 13.1), or there may be a large nodule which persists for many months.

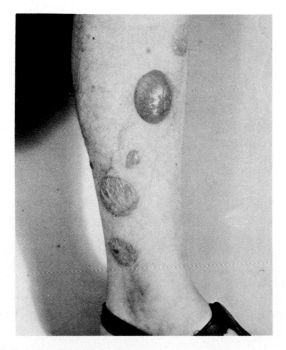

Fig. 13.1 Bullous reaction to insect bites

The histology of insect bites is very varied, and reflects the different immune responses. These may be a dense lymphocytic infiltrate, or there may be many plasma cells or eosinophils. There may be vasculitis, granuloma formation or even an epidermal proliferation which mimics squamous carcinoma (pseudo-epitheliomatous hyperplasia).

Treatment of insect bites

The source should if possible be removed. Insects on pets can be identified by brushing the animal on to a newspaper and sending the dander for microscopic examination by a zoologist. Dicophane powder (DDT) kills fleas in man, but the application of DDT to cats by well-meaning doctors has been known to provoke immediate licking of the area, with fatal results for the furry friend, and a noticeable cooling of the doctor-patient relationship.

If the source cannot be isolated insect repellants such as dimethylphthalate cream may be helpful. Oral antihistamines will reduce irritation, but local antihistamines should not be used as they are potent allergens and can cause severe dermatitis.

Fleas

The human flea (Pulex irritans) is a small brown insect renowned for its prodigious jumping power (a man-sized flea could jump over St. Paul's cathedral) (Fig. 13.2).

Flea-bites are a common cause of 'papular urticaria'. Many cats and dogs harbour fleas which will bite humans, but the reaction produced is very variable. The eggs are laid in crevices in floors or furniture, not on the host, and severe attacks may occur on moving

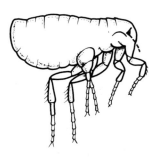

Fig. 13.2 Human flea

into empty premises previously occupied by infested pets. In this unfortunate circumstance, it may be advisable to buy a cat, which will 'suck up' the spare fleas like a vacuum cleaner.

Bed-bugs (Fig. 13.3)

These blood-sucking insects can live in cracks in furniture for long periods without food. Like fleas, they inflict 'papular urticaria' on unsuspecting humans.

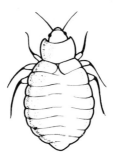

Fig. 13.3 Bed-bug

Lice

Lice are small, grey-brown, blood-sucking insects which crawl among the body hairs, and there are three distinct types according to the area infested (Fig. 13.4).

1. Pediculus capitis, the head louse
2. Pediculus corporis, the body louse
3. Phthirus pubis, the pubic louse, or 'crab'.

They are often difficult to find because they are translucent when not engorged with blood, but each female lays many eggs which are readily recognised as small white *nits*, each firmly attached to a hair shaft (Fig. 13.5).
Each nit hatches within 10 days.

1. Head lice

These occur in the long hair of the scalp, but may also invade eyebrows and eyelashes. They usually cause persistent irritation of the scalp, often with impetigo and occipital lymphadenopathy. Head lice have become common in recent years due to the emergence of

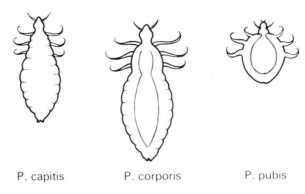

P. capitis   P. corporis   P. pubis

Fig. 13.4 Lice

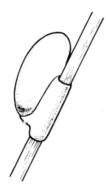

Fig. 13.5 Nit attached to hair

the so-called 'super-louse' which is resistant to DDT powder. Modern preparations such as 0.5 per cent malathion lotion are usually effective but contacts should also be treated. This will often involve treating a whole class of school-children.

Nits may be removed with a special fine-toothed metal comb, or the malathion application may be repeated 2 weeks later, when the larvae have hatched out.

2. Body lice

When not feeding, these live in the clothing, and the seams of underpants etc. must be searched carefully for nits. 'Vagabond's itch' is usually due to body lice but some affected individuals remain asymptomatic. Lice on a cooling dead body will look for alternative lodgings, and doctors asked to certify death in a vagrant should be aware of this.

Disease transmitted by body lice in endemic areas include typhus and relapsing fever.

3. 'Crab' lice

These usually inhabit the ano-genital area, and are often transmitted by sexual contact. They cause severe itching, and patients may present with pruritus ani or pruritus vulvae (p. 193).

Myiasis

This is an infestation by the larvae (maggots) of flies such as warble-flies and bot-flies. The eggs are laid in neglected ulcers, which later 'crawl' with maggots. In previous generations maggots were applied by doctors to wounds to remove necrotic tissue.

Some tropical flies such as the tumbu fly lay eggs in healthy skin, and thus produce red furuncle-like swellings, each containing a larva which breathes through a small airhole in the 'boil'.

Bees, wasps and hornets

The stings of these insects cause immediate pain, redness and swelling. This usually subsides within a few hours, but the cumulative effect of multiple stings can be fatal, especially in infants or frail old people.

The venom is potentially antigenic and hypersensitivity may develop. Subsequent stings will then cause either a severe local reaction or 'anaphylactic shock' (p. 207). Such patients should (i) avoid exposure, (ii) carry sublingual isoprenaline and (iii) wear a Medic-Alert bracelet. Cautious hyposensitization following skin tests may help.

Ants

Many species will inflict multiple painful bites if they are disturbed, and fire ants, which occur in USA, have been known to attack unconscious subjects.

Beetles

Some species contain blistering fluids (e.g., cantharadin) which are released when the beetle is crushed on the skin.

Caterpillars

Some species are covered in hairs which on contact with human skin will cause urticaria or a maculopapular rash.

ARACHNIDA

Scabies

This is a contagious disease caused by infestation with a mite (acarus) called *Sarcoptes scabiei* (Fig. 13.6).

The female mite, which is just large enough to be visible to the naked eye, burrows into the epidermis, where she lays her eggs. The burrows, which are about 3 mm long, can be easily seen as grey, thread-like irregular lines. The scabies mite was discovered in 1634, and sketched in 1657, but such is medical progress that others could not repeat the feat, and scabies was thought to be 'humoral' until the end of the nineteenth century, when a prize of 300 French crowns was offered to anyone who could demonstrate the mite. After a fraudulent claim from a pharmacist, who substituted a cheese mite, the prize was eventually won by a junior doctor who showed that the mite can be found in the burrows, but not usually in the vesicles, papules or excoriations. The burrows can be more readily identified by dropping a blob of ink on the sus-

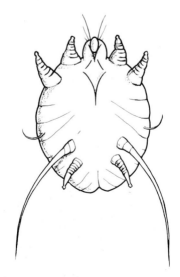

Fig. 13.6 Scabies mite

pected area and wiping it off with a moist swab. The burrow will then appear as a narrow dark line at one end of which may be a small pearly elevation containing the female mite. She can be unearthed by skilful probing with a needle at the end of the burrow, whence she may be transferred, still kicking, to a microscope slide for the education or edification of the patient or student. Male mites are rarely seen, since copulation causes their early demise.

The mite manifests itself clinically by causing severe pruritus, particularly when the patient is warm in bed. The burrows may be sparse, particularly in the well-washed, but there is usually a characteristic papular rash with multiple short excoriations. Burrows are most likely to be found between the fingers or on the flexor surface of the wrists. The papules are usually widespread (Fig. 13.7) but may be limited to the penis, buttocks, or around the areolae, i.e., sites which are likely to be overlooked during a hasty examination. The lesions do not occur above the neck-line. Most patients will recall contact with a similarly afflicted person, but the incubation period can be up to two months, since the pruritus does not occur until the individual has developed hypersensitivity to the mites or their excreta.

Though traditionally associated with the lower orders, scabies can occur in persons of irreproachable personal and moral hygiene. Experiments on 'conscientious objectors' which were precipitated by the epidemic of scabies during the 1939–45 war, showed that

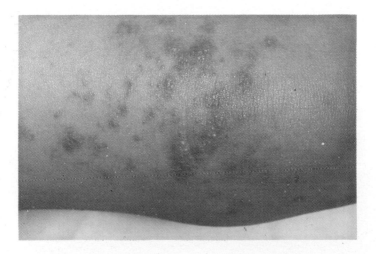

Fig. 13.7 Scabies

scabies was not readily transmitted by the bedding or underclothes used by infested patients, whereas prolonged bodily contact or the sharing of a bed readily transmitted the disease. This noble group summarized its conclusions as follows:

> Recondite research on Sarcoptes
> Has revealed that infections begin
> On leave with your wives and your children
> Or when you are living in sin.
> Except in the case of the clergy
> Who accomplish remarkable feats
> And catch scabies and crabs
> From door handles and cabs,
> And from blankets and lavatory seats.

Sexual promiscuity and overcrowding are not the only factors responsible for epidemics of scabies however, for these occur regularly in 30 year cycles, and it has been suggested that the 'herd immunity' of the population is more important than war-time conditions.

Treatment

Scabies is easy to cure, provided that patients are given (and follow) the correct advice. It is important that all members of the household and all close contacts (boyfriends etc.) should be treated simultaneously, otherwise reinfestation can readily cause an apparent 'failure of treatment'. Elderly members of the family can be asymptomatic reservoirs of infection and they often resent being treated. Treatment must be given on two consecutive nights, but not for longer, since anti-scabies preparations are primary irritants which will eventually cause eczema. This can be readily mistaken for active scabies, and the condition then becomes self-perpetuating.

The patient should first soak for 10 min in a warm bath, and this is followed by a brisk towelling to open the hydrated burrows. 1 per cent gamma benzene hexachloride cream is then applied to the whole body from the neck down, including the genitalia and the soles of the feet. This bathing and anointing is repeated on the second night, and on the following morning the patient has a complete change of bed-linen and underclothing, which is then laundered in the usual way. Patients should be warned that the pruritus may persist for a further 10 days, i.e., until the dead mites have been shed in the squames. Secondary eczematization of scabies is common, and anti-scabies preparations will then cause stinging, which is likely to result in inadequate application. Such patients are helped by the application of a steroid cream for a couple of days before the scabies is treated. Impetigo and lice should also be searched for and treated.

Norwegian scabies (Crusted scabies)

Norwegian scabies tends to occur in the mentally defective and the immuno-suppressed. It causes a somewhat psoriasiform rash which teems with mites and usually does not itch. Such cases are highly contagious, but they are rarely diagnosed until they have caused classical scabies in many contacts. The simultaneous occurrence of scabies in a doctor and a nurse may mean that they have shared nothing more exciting than a patient with Norwegian scabies.

Animal scabies ('Mange')

Mites which infest cats and dogs will occasionally invade humans, in whom they cause a puzzling irritable vesicular or urticated rash which mimics eczema or dermatitis herpetiformis. The rash clears following treatment of the animal and its bedding.

Food mites

Mites can sometimes be found in vast numbers in stored foods such as grain, flour and cheese. They can provoke either an urticated rash or allergic dermatitis in those handling the foodstuffs.

Ticks

These ectoparasites of many animals and man attach themselves firmly to the skin and suck blood for several days at a time. They cause no pain, but if the engorged spherical body of the tick is forcibly removed the mouth parts remain embedded. The judicious application of a lighted cigarette will induce the tick to release its victim. Another method is to cover the beast with a blob of nail varnish, when it will stop biting and gasp for air.

Spiders

A few foreign species are venomous. Black-widow spiders inject a powerful neurotoxin, and other species may cause severe local inflammation and necrosis by activation of the 'complement cascade' (p. 170). Contrary to popular belief the most dangerous spiders are small and shy, but they sometimes lurk beneath the rim of outdoor privies, which is a worrying thought.

C. OTHER NOXIOUS ANIMALS

The above catalogue by no means exhausts the sources of skin damage due to animals. Jelly fish stings and sea urchin spines may mar holidays. Cows' hooves regularly remove the skin from farmers' toes, and bull-fighters and postmen have their problems too, but the most noxious animal of all is the human.

Human bites, provoked by agony or by ecstasy, are particularly dangerous since the teeth harbour a variety of bacterial pathogens. Hands damaged by teeth during the administration of a 'knuckle sandwich' can develop tenosynovitis or even osteomyelitis if not adequately treated with surgical debridement and broad-spectrum antibiotics.

14

Ultra-violet radiation and the skin

The sun emits a continuous spectrum of electromagnetic energy from the short cosmic rays to the long radio waves (Fig. 14.1).

The ozone in the upper atmosphere provides a barrier to wavelengths shorter than 290 nm and so the earth's surface is shielded from the shorter wavelengths, which are inimical to most forms of life. The 'sunlight' which reaches ground level therefore consists of ultraviolet radiation (UVR) from 290 to 400 nm, and visible radiation from 400 to 700 nm.

Sunburn in humans is normally produced by a narrow band of radiation which extends only from 290 to 315 nm (UVB) (Fig. 14.2).

Shorter UV wavelengths (UVC) are more effective in burning the skin but they do not reach sea-level, though they do reach the peaks of high mountains, and they are emitted by some artificial light sources, e.g., 'bactericidal lamps'. The longer UV wavelengths (UVA) have relatively little effect on normal skin, and are invisible to man (though some insects can see UVA, which is reflected from flower petals in patterns which aid pollination and feeding by acting as a 'fight path' for the insect). The UVA wavelengths, sometimes

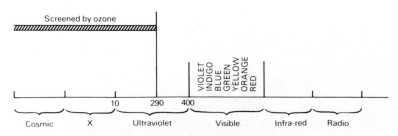

Fig. 14.1 Wavelengths (nanometres) emitted from sun's surface (not to scale). 1 nanometer is 1 millionth of a millimetre

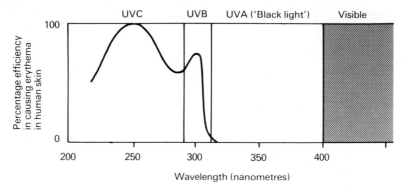

Fig. 14.2 Action spectrum for sunburn

called 'black light', are important in some diseases such as porphyria (p. 162), and drugs such as psoralens will sensitize the normal skin to UVA. Most window glass will absorb wavelengths shorter than 315 nm, and thus prevent sunburn, but patients with diseases which cause photosensitivity to 'black light' (UVA) can be badly burnt through glass.

A. EFFECTS OF SOLAR RADIATION ON NORMAL SKIN

1. Acute effects

(i) Erythema

Following exposure to UVB there is a latent period of 6 to 10 hr before the erythema develops. The minimal erythema dose (MED), which is used clinically to measure individual sensitivity, is the dose of a particular wavelength which is just sufficient to cause erythema in skin which has not recently been irradiated. With doses greatly in excess of the minimal erythema dose the latent period is decreased, and the victim may exhibit the well-known 'boiled-lobster' appearance within 2 hr. In severe sunburn there may be oedema and blistering, with nausea, vomiting, headache, rigors and even death. During recovery from sunburn there is widespread desquamation and pruritus. Prostaglandins are produced in the skin in sunburn, and indomethacin, which inhibits the prostaglandin synthetase enzyme, decreases the sunburn response to UVB irradiation.

UVA can cause erythema, but the dose required is very much greater.

Treatment of sunburn

'Prevention is better than cure', yet people who burn readily are caught out year after year because they fail to realize that

1. No discomfort is felt at the time of the irradiation, especially if there is a wind, which, by some unknown mechanism, actually increases sunburn

2. The sun's rays are most potent when the sun is overhead, i.e., at mid-day

3. Water, sand and snow reflect UVR and greatly increase the dose reaching the skin

4. Cloud cover and even thin clothing does not always form an impenetrable barrier to UVR

5. Sun-tan oils do not withstand prolonged or repeated immersion in water

Most greasy suntan preparations offer good protection from UVB irradiation. A useful liquid preparation which gives relatively long protection because it binds to the keratin layer of the epidermis is 2.5 per cent padimate (Spectraban). Topical sunscreening agents are now graded from 1 to 15 by a UVB 'protection factor', the higher numbers giving more protection.

For established sunburn, cooling lotions such as calamine are soothing, and in more severe cases topical steroids or even prednisone may be used.

(ii) Tanning

Both UVB and UVA appear to stimulate the formation of melanin for some days following exposure. The new melanin forms a 'cap' over the keratinocyte nuclei to protect the DNA from further damage.

(iii) Epidermal thickening

The epidermis may double its thickness following irradiation and this is probably as important as tanning in providing protection against future damage from UVR.

(iv) Vitamin D production

Vitamin D_3 (cholecalciferol) is formed in the skin by the UVB irradiation of dehydrocholesterol. Vitamin D_2 is taken in the diet but when this is deficient, exposure to sunlight will prevent rickets and osteomalacia. Elderly people often lack dietary D_2 and cannot get outdoors, and recent work suggests that the incidence of femoral neck fracture (which is associated with osteoporosis and histological osteomalacia) in the elderly might be reduced by increasing their exposure to UVR.

(v) Immunological effects

It is now well-established that PUVA therapy causes a temporary suppression of type 4 delayed hypersensitivity reactions in the skin. This is associated with a depletion of the epidermal Langerhans cells, which normally recognize antigens presented to the skin surface. The success of PUVA in treating cutaneous T cell lymphoma (p. 101) suggests that the irradiation also affects the lymphocytes. Recent work suggests that ordinary sunburn, without ingestion of a psoralen drug, can also produce immunosuppression. The implications of this work with regard to systemic infection has yet to be assessed, although in a previous generation, patients with tuberculosis were sometimes advised to avoid sunbathing as this was thought to exacerbate the infection.

2. Chronic effects

(i) 'Ageing' of skin,1

Many of the changes which we associate with ageing of the skin e.g., wrinkling, solar elastosis (p. 79), telangiectasis and lentigines are largely due to chronic exposure to UVR, and occur at an earlier age in sunny climates. There is some evidence that UVA can potentiate the damaging effect of the UVB wavelengths. This may be of importance in view of the growing trend for people to attend UVA solaria to 'top-up' their tans.

(ii) Solar keratoses (actinic keratoses)

These are premalignant scaly lesions which develop on skin damaged by UVR. In the UK they usually occur on the back of the hands, forehead or ear in elderly patients but in tropical countries 'sun-worshippers' may become vitually covered with keratoses in middle life. Clinically they form scaly, hyperpigmented plaques which may itch or ulcerate. The histology shows dysplastic changes, with loss of the normal keratinocyte maturation and areas of parakeratosis.

There is usually a period of several years between the development of a a solar keratosis and its transformation to squamous carcinoma, but the lesions should nevertheless be treated, particularly in younger patients.

Solar keratoses are best treated by cauterization or freezing. Topical 5-fluorouracil can also be used, but this produces a severe inflammatory reaction which causes discomfort for several weeks.

Patients with solar keratoses should be advised to avoid the sun, and to apply a topical sunscreen whenever exposure is unavoidable.

(iii) *Cutaneous malignancy* (p. 97).

All the chronic changes produced by UVR are less common in Negroes and more common in those with a Celtic complexion. Skin types can be classified according to their reaction to UVR as follows:

Type 1. Always burn, never tan.
Type 2. Always burn, sometimes tan.
Type 3. Sometimes burn, sometimes tan.
Type 4. Sometimes burn, always tan.
Type 5. Never burn, always tan.

The more sensitive types should take care to avoid the burning, ageing, immunosuppressive, carcinogenic rays, and should remain 'pale and interesting'.

B. PHOTODERMATOSES

These are skin diseases that are caused by an abnormal response to UV or visible radiation. They are usually recognized either by the history of sun-provocation, or by their distribution in the light-exposed areas.

1. Polymorphic light eruption

This is the commonest photodermatosis. It is a chronic disease of unknown aetiology, which commonly affects young women. Symptoms start in the spring, with itchy papules on light-exposed areas and the lesions often recur in crops until the autumn. Treatment is with topical sun-screening agents.

2. Photosensitivity due to drugs.

Many drugs induce photosensitivity, either as a dose-dependent effect (e.g., psoralens) or as an allergic response. The rash often resembles a chronic scaly eczema confined to light exposed areas, with a sharp 'cut-off' at the V of the neck, sleeves, etc. and it tends to spare the area beneath the chin. The following drugs are known photosensitizers:

(i)   Phenothiazines e.g., chlorpromazine
(ii) Thiazide diuretics
(iii) De-methyl-chlortetracycline
(iv) Tolbutamide and chlorpropamide
(v)   Nalidixic acid (this characteristically causes large blisters).

3. Photosensitivity due to external allergens

(i) Topical applications

Various chemicals added to soap and perfumes are photosensitizers, and the rash appears only in the light-exposed area. The diagnosis is confirmed by 'photo-patch' testing i.e., after application of a patch test in the usual way (p. 180) the area is irradiated, using a second non-irradiated patch as a control.

(ii) Airborne allergens

Dermatitis which is exacerbated by exposure to light is sometimes due to sensitization to plants of the Compositae family (chrysanthemum, etc). The allergen can occur in the pollen and, in India, a weed called Parthenium has been responsible for devastating attacks of light-sensitive erythroderma, since its pollen is as hard to avoid as grass-pollen is in Britain. In many patients the dermatitis can persist for months or even years after obvious exposure to the allergen has ceased, and such patients are called 'persistent light reactors'.

(iii) Actinic reticuloid

This is a severe and chronic form of photodermatitis which occurs in middle-aged or elderly men. It takes its name from the fact that the histology shows a very dense lymphocytic infiltrate in the dermis which resembles a lymphoma (hence 'reticuloid'), but the condition rarely, if ever, becomes malignant. The rash produces a characteristic cobblestone appearance on the back of the neck, and it often spreads to the covered parts, so that neither the patient nor his doctor may be aware of the provocative role of actinic irradiation. In some cases UVA from fluorescent lamps and even visible radiation can provoke the dermatitis.

Some of these patients seem to be 'persistent light reactors' following the development of allergy to plants or after-shave lotion. The patient is therefore condemned to lead a wretched and literally gloomy existence, avoiding daylight and even strong artificial light. Orange plastic window screens and 'barrier'-type sunscreen ointments may help, and in severe cases azathioprine may suppress the condition.

4. Porphyria

The porphyrias are a group of rare metabolic diseases in which excessive quantities of porphyrins or their precursors are produced. The diagnosis is made by finding these chemicals in the blood, urine or faeces. Enzyme deficiencies have been identified in every type.

(i) Acute intermittent porphyria (AIP)

This usually presents with abdominal pain and constipation or neuropsychiatric manifestations. The attacks are often precipitated by oestrogens, barbiturates or griseofulvin. Patients with AIP are recognized by the fact that their urine turns dark on standing. The skin is not affected.

(ii) Porphyria cutanea tarda (PCT)

Liver disease seems to precipitate this disease in genetically predisposed subjects, and most patients are middle-aged alcoholic men. The bald scalp and the backs of the hands develop haemorrhagic blisters on light-exposure. These crust over, and heal slowly to leave depressed scars. The skin is often fragile, and hypertrichosis and pigmentation are common.

Most patients have a raised plasma iron, with increased iron stores in the liver. A deficiency in hepatic uroporphyrinogen decarboxylase activity is probably present before the onset of the liver disease. Remove of the surplus iron by repeated venesections usually reduces the porphyrin production and dramatically improves the skin. Hydrochloroquine therapy is also effective, but it is important that the patient should avoid alcohol, or the condition will recur.

(iii) Erythro-hepatic protoporphyria (EPP)

In this type, photosensitivity develops in childhood, with redness and swelling of the exposed skin. A burning pain in the skin which is relieved by plunging the affected area under cold water is characteristic, but many of these patients have in the past been labelled neurotic. One of my colleagues made the diagnosis in a milkman who gained relief on summer mornings only by dousing his hands with milk. Oral β-carotene seems to be an effective treatment. Other porphyrins exist, but they are exceptionally rare in Britain. In South Africa a type called variegate porphyria, with features of AIP and PCT, is relatively common.

5. **Xeroderma pigmentosum** *(p. 96)*

C. SKIN DISEASES AGGRAVATED BY SUNLIGHT

Several other skin diseases are exacerbated or provoked by sunlight:

1. Herpes simplex
2. Lupus erythematosus
3. Rosacea.

D. SKIN DISEASES HELPED BY SUNLIGHT

1. *Psoriasis* is usually helped by UVR and this is an important method of treatment, but occasional patients react adversely.
2. *Acne vulgaris* usually benefits from UVR providing an erythema dose is used, but exceptional patients deteriorate.
3. *Eczema* often responds well to UVR, but some patients deteriorate. A few patients with constitutional eczema develop a super-imposed photosensitivity in later life.
4. *Venous leg ulcers* appear to be helped by UVR, which is said to decrease secondary infection and promote healing.

Considering that sunlight has been used as a therapeutic modality for thousands of years, we know disgustingly little about the way it acts in these four common diseases.

PROTECTION AGAINST SOLAR IRRADIATION

If a patient is suspected to be suffering from a photodermatosis, it is helpful if phototesting can be performed with a monochromator.

apparatus to determine the responsible wavelengths and the action spectrum. This may direct attention to specific causal agents (drugs, porphyrins, etc.) and will help in the choice of the most suitable sunscreening preparation.

Total protection is not always necessary. A regimen of graded exposure may help to develop the patient's own protective factors, and some cases (e.g., polymorphic light eruption) may benefit from pre-seasonal PUVA, UVB or phototherapy.

Many sunscreens are available, but they are mainly based on the following compounds:

(i) *Cinnamates*, or *para-aminobenzoic acid* and its *esters*. These protect against UVB.

(ii) *Benzophenones*. These protect against both UVB and UVA.

(iii) *Titanium dioxide* (a physical barrier). This protects against UVB, UVA and light.

15

Urticaria, angio-oedema and vasculitis

URTICARIA ('Hives')

This is a transient reaction characterized by dermal swelling due to vasodilatation and increased vascular permeability. It is recognised clinically as an itchy, blotchy, papular, erythematous rash, often with some central pallor. Each patch fades within 48 hr, leaving no trace, but new patches often develop at other sites.

Mechanisms of production

Urticaria can be produced by a wide variety of physical, chemical and immunological stimuli. It may be reproduced experimentally by the intra-dermal injection of *histamine* which produces the Lewis 'triple response' (erythema, oedema and surrounding axon flare), but many other vaso-active mediators such as kinins may be involved in producing clinical urticaria. Histamine is liberated by the degranulation of mast-cells, and this effect may be induced by several allergic and pharmacological mechanisms.

Some unusual types of urticaria which respond poorly to antihistamines may show histological evidence of vasculitis, with endothelial swelling and infiltration of the vessel wall by inflammatory cells. Red cells as well as plasma may escape into the dermis so that both urticaria and purpura may be seen. In more severe types of vasculitis there may be complete thrombosis of the vessel, with fibrinoid necrosis of its walls. There may thus be a spectrum of vascular damage ranging from normality to necrosis (Fig. 15.1).

Clinical types of urticaria

1. Acute urticaria

This is a common skin reaction which sooner or later affects at least 10 per cent of the population. It is sometimes the result of a Type

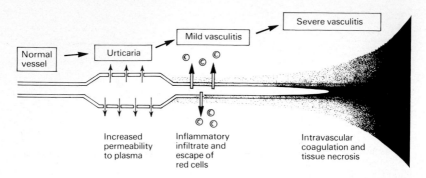

Fig. 15.1 The spectrum of vascular damage

1 allergic reaction (p. 207) to an ingested or injected antigen such as a specific food (e.g., nuts) or drug (e.g., penicillin) but often the cause cannot be identified. The condition is not invariably due to allergy. Some foods such as shellfish and strawberries can stimulate histamine release non-specifically, and other foods such as tuna fish and fermented cheeses are themselves a rich source of histamine. The response to anti-histamines may be poor, but most cases resolve spontaneously within a few weeks.

Occasionally urticated weals may be the presenting manifestation of another dermatosis such as dermatitis herpetiformis, pemphigoid, vasculitis or lupus erythematosus. They also occur occasionally in infantile eczema.

2. Chronic urticaria

Acute urticaria which has failed to resolve after an arbitrary period of about two months may be re-classified as chronic urticaria. These cases present a problem, since it is often difficult to identify the causative agent.

Aspirin sometimes provokes urticaria by a pharmacological mechanism and patients must be quizzed about the tablets they take for headaches, 'period pains' etc. Prostaglandin E_2 inhibits histamine release from mast cells, and it is thought that aspirin, which blocks prostaglandin synthesis, thus prevents this inhibition. *Candida* infection, which may be asymptomatic in the mouth, may also be a trigger for urticaria. A marked eosinophilia should suggest the possibility of an occult *parasite* such as a liver fluke infestation.

Preservatives (e.g., sodium benzoate) or *dyes* (e.g., tartrazine) in food-stuffs may also cause chronic urticaria, and these can be identified by 'challenge tests' in which the patient is given an oral dose of each of the possible culprits on successive days, interspersed by control tablets. A carefully-kept food diary may occasionally be helpful, and if this gives a clue, then a special elimination diet may provide confirmation. Skin testing is rarely useful, since it is bedevilled with false positives and false negatives, and many patients with urticaria respond even to the control tests.

Anthistamines will provide partial or complete relief for most patients, but it is often necessary to gradually increase the dose and alter the time of administration until the urticaria is suppressed or side-effects exceed the therapeutic benefit. The traditional antihistamines such as chlorpheniramine maleate and mepyramine maleate almost always cause drowsiness, especially in high doses, but the newer antihistamines terfenadine, oxatomide and astemizole seem not to cause this side-effect.

The skin microvasculature contains both H1 and H2 receptors for histamine and if the traditional H1 antihistamines alone are ineffective, the addition of an H2 blocker such as cimetidine may be helpful.

3. Physical urticaria

This is a distinctive group of diseases in which weals occur in response to physical stimuli.

(i) Dermographism

In this condition firm stroking of the skin causes an exaggerated 'triple response' (Fig. 15.2) so that messages can be transmitted on the skin in urticated letters. Dermographism occurs in 5 per cent of the population, and the tendency may persist indefinitely.

Symptomatic dermographism is associated with severe itching. It occurs mainly in young adults and may resolve spontaneously within a few months.

Many doctors confuse dermographism with chronic urticaria, but the incidence of dermographism in chronic urticaria is the same as in the general population.

(ii) Pressure urticaria

In this rare condition, which is unrelated to dermographism, sustained pressure, (e.g., on the buttocks), causes deep painful swell-

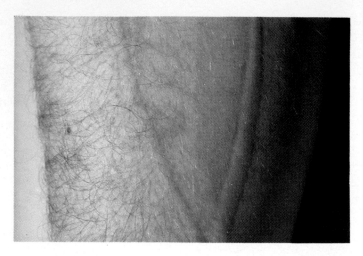

Fig. 15.2 Dermographism

ings which develop after a delay of some hours and persist for 24 to 48 hours.

(iii) Cold urticaria

Wealing of the skin on exposure to cold may occur as an idiopathic condition, or it may be secondary to diseases, such as myeloma, lupus erythematosus and syphilis, which produce cryoglobulins or cold haemolysins. In cold urticaria collapse due to massive histamine release may follow sudden immersion in cold water (e.g., sea-bathing). Tolerance can be induced by repeated exposure to cold showers, but the cure is probably worse than the disease.

(iv) Local heat urticaria and solar urticaria

In these rare conditions exposure to local heat or ultra-violet radiation respectively provokes urticaria.

4. Cholinergic urticaria (micro-papular urticaria)

This is a very distinctive condition in which a crop of extremely irritable small weals develops after sweating, whether induced by heat, exercise, emotion or hot spicy foods. Mild forms of this disease are not uncommon, especially in young adults. Antihistamines such as hydroxyzine are usually more helpful than anti-cholinergic drugs, but after each attack there is a refractory period for 12 to 24 hours, and some patients prefer to take a hot bath to give themselves immunity for subsequent activities likely to involve heat, exercise and emotion.

5. Papular urticaria (p. 147)

6. Urticaria pigmentosa

In this rare condition there is a widespread patchy accumulation of mast cells in the skin. It usually develops during childhood, but the onset is occasionally delayed to adult life. The abnormal skin can be recognised as yellowish-brown macules or papules which urticate and itch when they are rubbed. In about one third of cases there may also be involvement of the bone, liver and spleen (systemic mastocytosis).

A mast-cell naevus is a similar condition in which a congenital accumulation of mast cells is localized to one area of the skin.

ANGIO-OEDEMA ('GIANT URTICARIA')

This is a variant of urticaria which affects the subcutaneous tissues rather than the dermis, but there is often a considerable overlap between the two conditions. Angio-oedema commonly affects the lips and the peri-orbital tissue (Fig. 15.3). In the latter site it is easily mistaken for contact dermatitis due to an air-borne allergen (e.g., hair-spray), but angio-edema, unlike dermatitis, does not cause scaling of the eye-lids.

Hereditary angio-oedema

This is a rare but important disease, transmitted as an autosomal dominant, which causes recurrent deep swellings of the skin and mucous membranes, often after minimal trauma. Involvement of the gastro-intestinal tract causes nausea, vomiting and colic and some patients have been subjected to repeated laparotomies by keen surgeons. Laryngeal involvement causes respiratory obstruction and the patient may die of asphyxiation unless tracheostomy is performed.

These patients lack a specific Cl-esterase inhibitor, which normally keeps the 'complement cascade' in check (Fig. 15.4). Any stimuli which activate complement therefore initiate a complex train

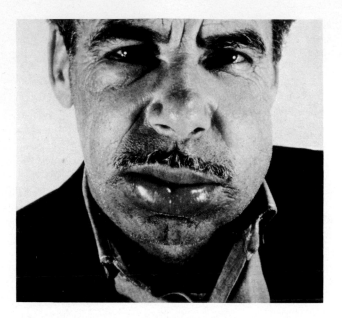

Fig. 15.3 Angio-oedema of the mouth and right periorbital area

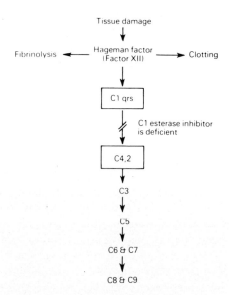

Fig. 15.4 The complement cascade in hereditary angio-oedema

of reactions which result in massive liberation of kinins. Anabolic steroids such as danazol have a very beneficial effect in preventing the attacks, probably by boosting the synthesis of the deficient protein in the liver.

VASCULITIS

Vasculitis is a taxonomic imbroglio, which is to say that its classification is a mess. Patients with vasculitis may be classified according to their clinical features, their histological features, (size of vessel, type of infiltrate, etc.) or their immunological features (immunoglobulin and complement levels, type of immune complex, etc.), but unfortunately the correlation between the three methods is poor, and whichever is used, some patients cannot be neatly categorized.

Vasculitis in the skin may present a wide variety of clinical appearances, including urticaria, livedo reticularis (p. 89), purpura, macules, papules, pustules, haemorrhagic blisters, necrotic ulcers and scars, but these features do not occur simultaneously, and often only one type of lesion is present.

Cutaneous vasculitis occurs in the following conditions:

1. Polyarteritis nodosa

This is a serious but uncommon disease in which a patchy necrotizing inflammation develops in many medium-sized arteries throughout the body. The hepatitis B virus has been shown to provoke the disease in some patients, but often no cause can be found. Middle-aged men are the usual victims. There is usually a systemic illness, with fever, malaise, tachycardia, leucocytosis and a high ESR or plasma viscosity.

The skin changes may include:
(i)   Small nodules which occur along the course of superficial arteries
(ii) Livedo reticularis
(iii) Purple necrotic plaques, haemorrhagic bullae or deep 'punched-out' ulcers with an irregular margin (Fig. 15.5).

Any internal organ may be involved, and common complications include hypertension, renal failure, myocardial ischaemia, gastrointestinal bleeding, peripheral neuropathy and focal cerebral lesions.

The prognosis is variable, but some patients deteriorate rapidly despite treatment with prednisone and immunosuppressive drugs.

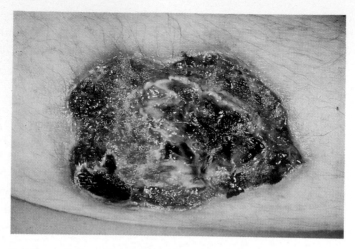

Fig. 15.5 Necrosis due to polyarteritis nodosa

Cases with pulmonary involvement (asthma, haemoptysis and pneumonitis) and a circulating eosinophilia appear to form a subgroup with a good prognosis. Occasionally polyarteritis nodosa is confined to the skin and these patients also do well.

2. Cranial arteritis ('giant cell' arteritis)

This is a disease of the elderly which predominantly affects the temporal arteries. It causes fever, and severe headache, with tender red nodules along the superficial cranial arteries. The ESR is often very high. Visual loss is common, and early treatment with large doses of prednisone may be needed to prevent blindness. The scalp may blister and become necrotic, and the condition is then readily confused with herpes zoster.

3. Wegener's granulomatosis

This is a rare but often fatal disease, which is characterized by granulomatous necrosis of the upper or lower respiratory tract, with widespread necrotizing arteritis and severe glomerulonephritis. Patients usually present with persistent bleeding and ulceration of the nostrils. Signs of cutaneous vasculitis occur in about 50 per cent of cases.

4. Leukocytoclastic ('allergic') vasculitis

This is a histological diagnosis. The inflammation affects small vessels (often venules) and there is a marked peri-vascular infiltrate with many fragmented polymorphs ('nuclear dust') and a variable number of eosinophils. Allergy to drugs or micro-organisms is often blamed for this disease, often without much evidence. Many clinical patterns have been described and dignified by eponyms, but this rarely helps in management. In many cases the lesions are confined to the skin (Fig. 15.6), and local factors such as stasis and cold determine the distribution of the lesions. Purpura of the lower legs is common, and many patients improve with bed rest. Dapsone orally is helpful in some cases, but in the more severe cases which do not respond to dapsone, systemic prednisone may be needed.

Henoch-Schönlein purpura, which was first described by an Englishman called Smith, is a type of leukocytoclastic vasculitis which occurs predominantly in children. The syndrome comprises an urticated or purpuric rash, flitting arthralgia, gastro-intestinal symptoms (pain, vomiting and bloody diarrhoea) and a focal proliferative glomerulonephritis. The prognosis depends on the degree of renal damage, but most patients recover. Vasculitis is a common feature of the 'collagen-vascular' diseases, especially rheumatoid disease (see Chapter 20).

5. Erythema nodosum

This nodular eruption, which mainly affects young adults, is usually confined to the lower legs (Fig. 15.7), though it occasionally affects the thighs or forearms. In a typical case 5 to 10 large, red,

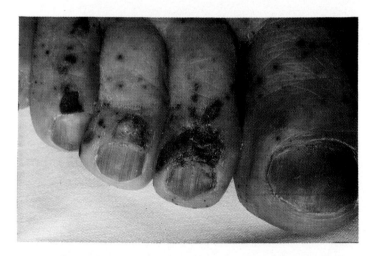

Fig. 15.6 Leukocytoclastic vasculitis

oval, raised patches, hot and tender to palpation, erupt over a period of about 10 days. There is often fever, malaise and arthralgia, which almost always affects the knees. In the second or third week the inflammation begins to subside and the lesions go through the same sequence of colour changes as a fading bruise (purple, brown, yellowish-green). The skin lesions resolve in 3 to 6 weeks, although the arthralgia may be more persistent.

The condition is an immunological reaction to a variety of precipitating causes, including sarcoidosis, tuberculosis, streptococcal infection, sulphonamides, viruses and bedsoniae. Circulating immune-complexes have been found in some cases, and though the histology is non-specific, there may be a mild vasculitis in the lower dermis and upper fat layer.

6. Other nodular forms of cutaneous vasculitis

There are several other conditions (e.g., Bazin's disease) affecting the lower legs, which are characterised by chronic or recurrent nodules, varying degrees of vasculitis and a tendency to ulceration. They are not clearly defined however, and until our immu-knowhow improves they may be conveniently labelled as 'nodular vasculitis'.

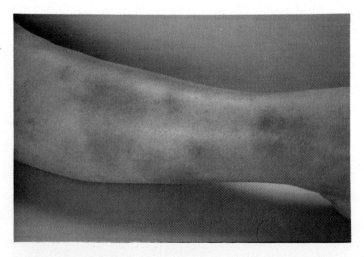

Fig. 15.7 Erythema nodosum

16

Eczema

Eczema is a particular pattern of inflammatory response in the skin, of which spongiosis (epidermal oedema) is the hallmark. It may be induced by both external and internal factors acting singly or in combination. The terms dermatitis and eczema are now used synonymously, although in the past some dermatologists have restricted the term dermatitis to an eczematous reaction due to an occupational cause.

Clinical features

The clinical presentation of eczema is variable but fairly distinctive. The cardinal symptom is itching, which may be very severe. The cardinal signs are redness, papules, vesicles, hyperkeratosis with scaling, exudation of serum ('weeping') and crusting. None of these features is specific to eczema and they do not always occur together, but nevertheless the combination of these signs usually makes eczema readily recognizable to the dermatologist. Fungal infection is perhaps the condition which is most likely to be mistaken for eczema, but in fungal infection the edge of the rash is well-demarcated (unless steroid ointments have been applied) whereas eczema is more diffuse.

Pathology

Eczema may be acute, sub-acute or chronic and the histology and clinical appearance vary in the different stages (Fig. 16.1).

1. Acute eczema

Acute eczema predominantly affects the epidermis and uppermost (papillary) part of the dermis. The first histological sign of eczema

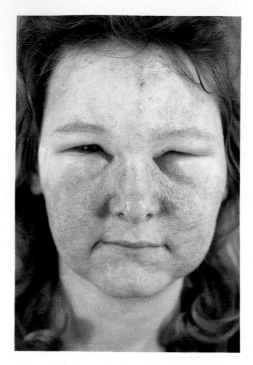

Fig. 16.1 Acute contact dermatitis due to cosmetic allergy

is the development of epidermal oedema (*spongiosis*). Extracellular fluid accumulation causes separation of the prickle cells so that the intercellular bridges become prominent, and intracellular oedema causes the cells to become swollen and rounded.

The change occurs irregularly along the epidermis, starting as discrete foci in the mid-epidermal region, but as it becomes more severe, the oedematous areas coalesce to form clinical vesicles. As the pressure increases, fluid leaks on to the surface and the skin 'weeps'. The serous fluid mixed with cellular debris then coagulates to form yellowish 'crusts'. In regions with a tough horny layer, such as the palms and soles, the vesicles rupture less readily, and large bullae (up to 2 cm in diameter) may form. In these areas, the vesicles often look like deep-seated sago grains, with little erythema. In other areas, the dermal blood-vessels become dilated and the capillary permeability is increased. There is usually a dermal infiltrate composed mainly of lymphocytes, but in some cases polymorphs and red cells also accumulate.

2. Sub-acute and chronic eczema

As eczema becomes more chronic, the oedema tends to diminish, and *acanthosis* (an increased thickness of the prickle cell layer) develops (Fig. 16.2). At the same time, due to the disturbance of normal keratinization, there is *parakeratosis* (retention of nuclei in the horny layer) and *hyperkeratosis* (increased thickness of the horny layer) (Fig. 16.3).

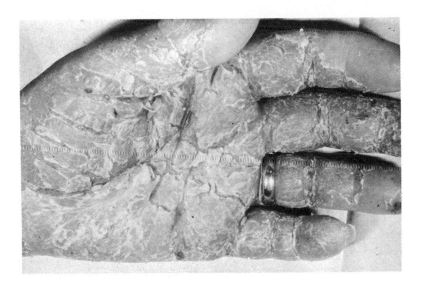

Fig. 16.2 Subacute hand eczema

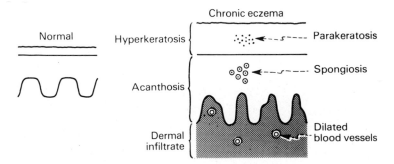

Fig. 16.3 Histology of eczema

The increased thickness of the epidermis with the underlying oedema and infiltrate produces areas of skin in which the normal skin lines become greatly exaggerated, so that the skin looks rather like the bark of a tree (Fig. 16.4). This change, which is called *lichenification*, is often associated with severe itching and it is particularly common in atopic subjects (p. 183). In chronic eczema the vascular dilatation gradually becomes less marked, but the dermal lymphocytic infiltrate often persists, particularly around the vessels.

Secondary spread

Eczema shows a characteristic tendency to spread widely from its point of origin. This may occur by direct extension of the affected area, or new patches may appear in a completely different area. The mechanism of this dissemination is obscure, but some cases are undoubtedly due to a contact factor, either as a result of continued exposure to the initial allergen, or secondary to the development of sensitivity to a topical medicament.

AETIOLOGY AND CLASSIFICATION OF ECZEMATOUS REACTIONS

This is a complex problem because many pathogenetic factors may be involved, and these are poorly understood. Eczema due to some external agent coming into contact with the skin is called *exogenous*

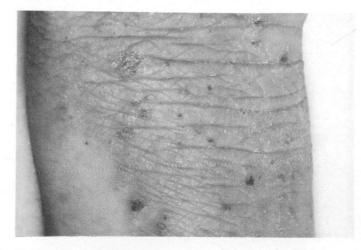

Fig. 16.4 Chronic lichenified eczema

dermatitis and all other cases are said to be *endogenous* (constitutional). In some cases however both constitutional and external factors may be important. Moreover the sub-classification of endogenous eczema depends on the clinical features and the various patterns may overlap. No completely reliable or rational classification exists, but the following guide may help.

Classification of eczema

A. Exogenous (i.e., due to an external factor)

1. Contact dermatitis
    (i) Primary irritant
    (ii) Allergic
2. Infective.

B. Endogenous (i.e., constitutional)

1. Atopic dermatitis
2. 'Seborrhoeic' dermatitis
3. Gravitational ('varicose') eczema
4. Asteatotic eczema
5. Discoid eczema
6. Hand eczema
7. Chronic superficial scaly dermatitis.

A. EXOGENOUS

1. Contact Dermatitis

(i) Primary irritant

A primary irritant is a substance which, if applied in high enough concentration to normal skin is capable of producing an eczematous response following a single exposure. Caustic liquids such as acids and alkalis are strong primary irritants, but of much more clinical importance are mild primary irritants such as detergents and mineral oils which may require prolonged contact to provoke eczema. A primary irritant will thus cause dermatitis in everyone if it is applied in sufficient concentration for a sufficient time. Repeated minor traumatization of the skin such as occurs in housework and in many industries can also provoke a 'wear and tear' eczema. These is however considerable variation in the degree of resistance to this type of damage in the normal population. It follows that many manual workers in dirty or wet conditions are at risk of developing hand eczema and it can be difficult in an individual case to assess how much of the damage is due to exogenous factors and how much is constitutional.

Napkin dermatitis ('nappy rash')

This primary irritant dermatitis occurs in babies due to prolonged contact with urine or faeces, sometimes as a result of ammonia production by bacteria. Conditions which favour its development include frequent loose stools, delay in napkin changing, inadequate cleaning of the buttocks or napkins, and occlusive rubber or plastic pants. The skin folds are usually spared, whereas the reverse is true of Candidosis.

Most cases of napkin dermatitis respond to improved hygiene and the application of an emollient or a silicone protective cream. In more severe cases Vioform HC cream is helpful, but potent steroids should not be used.

(ii) Allergic dermatitis ('hypersensitivity dermatitis')

This is due to the development of delayed hypersensitivity (Type 4 allergy) to a specific chemical, known as the *sensitizer* or *allergen*.

Such chemicals will not cause eczema even in high concentration in a normal person, but severe eczema may be provoked by brief exposure to a very low concentration of the chemical in a sensitized person. Chemicals vary in their capacity to provoke sensitization and the number of exposures required to produce sensitization varies correspondingly from a few to infinity.

There is probably also a variation in the genetic susceptibility of the individual to develop delayed hypersensitivity. A few chemicals such as dinitrochlorobenzene (DNCB) will eventually sensitize almost 100 per cent of normal people, but for most chemicals the risk is very much smaller. Some naturally-occurring substances such as uroshiol found in poison oak and poison ivy, are very potent sensitizers, and many people in North America develop severe reactions from these plants. Some chemicals of low molecular weight (e.g., nickel) can act as *haptens* i.e., they bind to a protein and the resulting complex then acts as an allergen.

In some cases it is easy to diagnose contact dermatitis from the distribution of the rash e.g., a band across the forehead from a leather hatband, or a small patch of eczema beneath a metal bra-fastener. More often the recognition of a contact allergy requires considerable patience and acumen (Fig. 16.5). According to the area affected the doctor may need to obtain a detailed history of the patient's occupation, household duties, hobbies, clothes, cosmetics and even contraceptives. In the case of occupational dermatitis a considerable knowledge of chemistry and industrial processes is required, and the doctor may have to visit the factory to observe the working conditions and to search for possible sensitizers. Patients sometimes develop contact dermatitis from a local preparation bought from the pharmacist, and a surprising number deny applying anything to the skin. In such intractable cases it is worth visiting the home and checking the contents of the bathroom cupboard, etc.

Virtually any chemical occasionally causes sensitivity, but the following are well known sensitizers in everyday use:

1. Metals, especially nickel and chromium. These occur in traces in jewellery, but they are found also in less likely places such as detergents (Ni) and cement (Cr)

2. Rubber, due to the accelerant and anti-oxidant chemicals used in its manufacture.

3. Organic dyes, especially paraphenylenediamine (PPD)

4. Plastics and resins e.g., spectacles and nail varnish

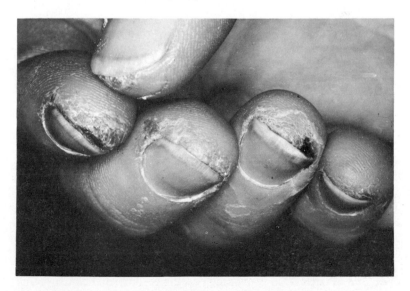

Fig. 16.5 Dermatitis of the fingertips due to handling tulip bulbs

5. Preservatives in ointments and cosmetics (e.g., parabens)
6. Plants, especially primula
7. Drugs applied topically, especially antihistamine creams (often sold for the treatment of insect bites), and local anaesthetic creams.

Many allergens may be difficult to eliminate from the environment, either because they are ubiquitous e.g., nickel in coins, cutlery and canned food, or because they occur in a variety of disguises, e.g., chromate occurs in cement, chrome steel, anticorrosive paint, tanned leather, green tattoo pigment, photographic chemicals, matches, fuel ashes, welding fumes and foundry sand.

Patch tests

Once a substance is suspected to be causing allergic contact dermatitis, it may be tested by applying it (preferably in solution) to an area of unaffected skin under a small patch of adhesive tape. The patch is removed at 48 hr, or earlier if severe irritation develops. A positive reaction consists of erythema, sometimes with swelling and vesiculation of the area.

This test is simple to perform, but its interpretation is fraught with pitfalls, of which three examples are given:

1. Some sensitizers are also primary irritants and they give a positive reaction in every patient unless they are suitably diluted
2. The positive response may not appear for 24 hr after the patch has been removed
3. A positive result does not necessarily mean that the substance is the cause of the eczema. The patient may be allergic to other substances, or may also have a constitutional eczema.

Nevertheless patch tests remain a very worthwhile investigation; both to confirm suspected allergies and to suggest possibilities (using a standard 'battery' of common sensitizers) which need further discussion with the patient.

Patch tests should be avoided when the eczema is in the acute phase, as a positive test can cause a severe exacerbation in all the affected areas.

2. Infective dermatitis

The role of bacteria in provoking eczema is somewhat controversial, but some cases of eczema with a positive culture occasionally respond to antibiotic therapy alone.

B. ENDOGENOUS ECZEMA ('Constitutional eczema')

1. Atopic eczema

Asthma, hay-fever, urticaria and infantile eczema tend to run in certain families, and sometimes two or more of these conditions may develop simultaneously or consecutively in the same person. The predisposition to these diseases is called the *atopic diathesis*, and it is present in about 10 per cent of the population.

The exact pathogenesis of atopic eczema is obscure, but atopic subjects tend to produce very high levels of circulating IgE (reaginic) antibodies which are involved in Type 1 hypersensitivity reactions. There is some evidence that infants with eczema have a low level of IgA secretion into the intestine, together with a deficiency of suppressor T cells, and the increased IgE may be secondary to these abnormalities. Dietary allergens, particularly cows' milk, may also play a part in provoking eczema, and babies from atopic families should be breast fed for at least three months as this has been shown to decrease the risk of eczema. Admittedly one large study showed that breast-fed babies have a higher than average incidence of atopic dermatitis, but this could be explained by the fact that well-informed mothers with a genetic tendency to atopy now make a special effort to breast-feed.

The value of dietary restriction (cows' milk, eggs, nuts, etc.) in the management of atopic eczema is a very controversial topic. Most British dermatologists feel that the possibility of food allergy should be tested by dietary exclusion and 'challenge' tests on one occasion, but if no definite allergic reaction is demonstrated, stringent dietary restrictions are not advisable. Various laboratory tests such as the radio-allergosorbent test (RAST) do not seem to provide reliable guidance in this situation.

Some atopic eczema patients have a decreased level of blood essential fatty acids, and this can be corrected by the oral ingestion of evening primrose oil, with clinical improvement in about 50 per cent of cases.

Atopic eczema is never present at birth but appears after a few weeks or more, and it may continue or recur in adult life. The face is often affected first (Fig. 16.6), but any area may be involved thereafter, particularly the knee and elbow flexures. Itching is often severe and the baby is often fretful because of this. The disease tends to wax and wane, and the long-term course is unpredictable but over 90 per cent will be clear by the age of 15 yr. Atopic eczema may be only a transient irritation or it may be a life-long disability which ruins the patient's life.

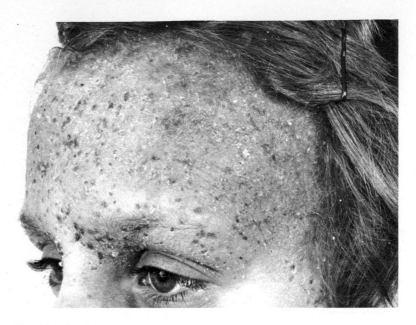

Fig. 16.6 Atopic eczema

Patients with atopic eczema tend to have a dry flaky skin (xeroderma). This dryness tends to exacerbate the itching, and the regular application of an emollient ointment, together with the prevention of over-frequent bathing (which paradoxically causes further drying of the skin) will often produce a dramatic improvement in the irritation. Excessive heat and woollen clothing also exacerbate atopic eczema, and afflicted babies should be dressed in cool cotton clothes.

Patients with atopic eczema should avoid exposure to herpes simplex and should not be vaccinated against smallpox because of the risk of Kaposi's varicelliform eruption (p. 118). Their immunity to other infective agents appears to develop in the normal way.

2. 'Seborrhoeic' eczema

'Seborrhoeic' eczema is recognized by its characteristic distribution, but the diagnostic criteria are somewhat nebulous, and dermatologists differ in their readiness to attach this diagnostic label. The term 'seborrhoeic' eczema is a misnomer, since many elderly patients with this condition have a dry skin. The condition probably has no special relationship to sebaceous glands, but old names die hard and new ones abort easily.

There are three main patterns of rash, which may occur in any combination:

(i) There is redness and diffuse scaling of the scalp (dandruff, pityriasis capitis) which may be mild or severe. Red scaly patches also occur on the face, especially in the eyebrows and the naso-labial folds. A similar rash occurs behind the ears, and otitis externa and blepharitis are common.

(ii) Small red patches with prominent scales occur on the trunk (Fig. 16.7). These tend to be localized over the sternum or the inter-scapular areas, especially in young men. There is little irritation, and in this situation the rash is sometimes mistaken for pityriasis rosea, psoriasis or even tinea corporis.

(iii) The body folds (axillae, groin, sub-mammary areas) become bright-red, moist and macerated, particularly in the middle-aged or elderly. This type of eczema, which occurs at sites of close skin apposition, is called *intertrigo*. There is often secondary invasion by Candida.

The pathogenesis of 'seborrhoeic' eczema is unknown. There is some evidence that severe dandruff is associated with an increased population of yeasts in the scalp, and if these are eradicated by an antiseptic shampoo e.g., cetrimide, the redness and scaling improves. It has been suggested that the abnormal proliferation of the normal skin flora predisposes to seborrhoeic eczema. Some patients with 'seborrhoeic' eczema are susceptible to boils, and it may be

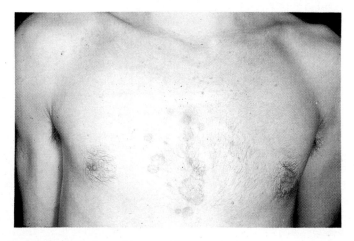

Fig. 16.7 Seborrhoeic dermatitis over the sternum

that such patients have a fundamental defect which allows skin flora to proliferate readily. Certain yeast-like organisms such as Pityrosporum ovale can activate the alternate complement pathway, and this might play a role in causing the cutaneous inflammation. The histology gives little clue to the aetiology, since it shows some features of both eczema and psoriasis.

3. Gravitational eczema ('varicose' eczema)

This is a distinctive pattern of eczema which develops in adult (usually elderly) patients with venous hypertension of the legs (p. 90). There is diffuse irritation, redness and scaling of the lower third of the leg, with a marked tendency to brown pigmentation. Most patients have obvious varicose veins and 'leashes' of blue venules are often visible over the dorsum of the foot and around the ankle.

Secondary spread of the eczema to other parts of the body is common, so that the diagnosis is missed if the legs are not examined. The development of *allergic sensitization* to topically applied medicaments (e.g., antibiotics) is also common in gravitational eczema.

4. Asteatotic eczema

This term refers to eczema which is secondary to epidermal lipid depletion. Elderly patients and patients with hypothyroidism or chronic renal failure often have a dry flaky skin, and this is associated with a tendency to itching and cracking of the skin, particularly in cold dry weather (i.e., 'chapping'). This distinctive clinical picture, with reticulate cracks and erythema (sometimes called 'eczèma craquelé') often responds well to simple emollients which prevent the keratin from cracking.

5. Discoid eczema

This is a poorly-understood pattern, characterized by well-demarcated disc-shaped areas of eczema. Discoid eczema commonly affects the extensor surfaces of the limbs in middle-aged adults.

6. Eczema of the palms and soles

Eczema of the palms and soles is a common condition which can be due to exogenous factors, but if no cause is identified the diagnosis of 'constitutional eczema' is made by exclusion.

Clinically there is diffuse redness and scaling, and because of the thick horny layer, there may be large blisters ('pompholyx'). Hyperkeratosis may be marked, with painful fissures which impair manual dexterity. This condition can be very intractable, but if it does not respond to the usual measures (p. 188), PUVA or superficial X-ray therapy may be helpful.

Hand eczema is often the result of several factors including an atopic tendency, dry skin, repeated exposure to mild irritants, repeated trauma, secondary infection, etc. and it can be difficult in medico-legal cases to apportion blame. In some industries dermatitis is so common as to be accepted as part of the job. Barrier creams are usually of very limited benefit, and patients are often reluctant to change their job for financial reasons.

Hand eczema may occur alone, or it may occur in association with any of the other patterns mentioned above. All areas should be examined, particularly the feet, in case the hand eczema is the result of a secondary spread or an 'ide' reaction. Other diseases which can cause diffuse redness and scaling of the palms and soles include fungal infection, psoriasis and lichen planus.

7. Chronic superficial scaly dermatitis (Benign parapsoriasis)

This eczematous process of unknown aetiology produces yellowish-pink oval flaky patches on the thighs and trunk, which have characteristic 'finger-like' extensions. Mild itching is common, and the disease is controlled, but not cured, by steroid ointments.

Management of eczema

The most important consideration is to identify and remove causative factors if possible. In allergic contact eczema this can be very difficult, and prolonged interrogation and investigation, including a visit to the patient's home and place of work may occasionally be required. Patients sometimes fail to identify the sensitizing chemical in their environment even when patch tests have proved positive.

The treatment of eczema varies at different stages.

Acute eczema which is vesicular and moist should be treated several times daily with potassium permanganate soaks diluted to a pink colour (about 1:8000). This is a soothing lotion which prevents secondary infection and tends to reduce the 'weeping', but it will cause dryness and cracking of the skin if continued for too long.

A steroid cream should be used to prevent inflammation, and in very severe and widespread cases, systemic prednisone may also be necessary. As the eczema recovers, a less potent steroid cream should be substituted.

Secondary bacterial infection should be treated with an appropriate systemic antibiotic, and many steroid creams are available with an added antimicrobial component. Patients should be warned that the commonly used antiseptic clioquinol causes yellow staining of white clothes. One of my colleagues incurred the wrath of a patient by advising the application of gentian violet to her infected eczematous baby, who subsequently left a serpentine purple trail over an expensive white carpet.

In *chronic eczema* it may be advisable to use a less water-soluble preparation. Patient preferences vary, but many atopics, and men with heavy jobs, prefer an ointment which is not readily absorbed but which greases the skin and protects it from external irritants. Other patients, particularly women, prefer a water-soluble cream which is absorbed and therefore feels less greasy.

In patients with the dry skin (xeroderma) of atopic eczema a simple emollient such as Aqueous Cream or Emulsifying Ointment will often relieve pruritus. Over-frequent bathing causes removal of skin lipids with consequent dehydration of keratin, and this makes eczema worse. Perfumed soaps are often irritant and should be replaced with Simple Soap, or by a liquid suspension of Emulsifying Ointment (1 tablespoonful mixed in a cup of very hot water).

Children with atopic eczema often lose sleep and become fretful because of the constant irritation. Woollens should not be worn next to the skin, but loose fitting cotton clothes are suitable. For babies, mitts may be needed to prevent excoriations. An antihistamine sedative such as trimeprazine tartrate syrup is often helpful, provided a big enough dose is used.

Topical steroids are the mainstay of suppressive treatment for chronic eczema, because of their undoubted efficacy and cosmetic acceptability. Patients should be warned of possible side-effects (p. 250), the weakest preparation effective for a particular patient should be used, and with the most potent steroids such as clobetasol propionate, patients should be followed-up as carefully as if they were taking systemic prednisone. Patients who have failed to respond to treatment as an outpatient will often improve dramatically when the same therapy is used following admission to hospital. Various *tar preparations*, e.g., White's Tar Paste, also help chronic eczema, but they are messier and less effective than glucocorticoids. Before the advent of glucocorticoids, sea bathing was the traditional remedy for eczema, and some patients still find it helpful to add salt to their bath-water. Other patients find oatmeal baths very soothing, but the use of hot porridge is not recommended.

JUVENILE PLANTAR DERMATOSIS

This condition is considered separately because it is debatable whether it is a true eczema. The term refers to the development of a scaly, glazed, fissured erythema on the weight-bearing parts of the fore-feet of school-children. The disease was rarely if ever seen before the 1960s, and it is believed to result from the increased use of impermeable plastics in footwear. It tends to occur in 'sporty' children who wear trainer shoes for prolonged periods every day (and in some cases, one suspects, all night too). Maceration of the skin, with blockage of the sweat ducts is probably an important factor. The response to steroid ointments is often poor, but many cases clear up if permeable leather shoes are worn. The condition clears spontaneously at puberty.

17

Pruritus

Pruritus (itching) is defined as a sensation which provokes the desire to scratch. It originates from stimulation of the subepidermal nerve plexus by a variety of agents, including histamine and various proteases, and their effect is enhanced by prostaglandins which are often present in inflamed skin. Several other vaso-active peptides which are released during the process of inflammation, induce pain rather than itch, and the precise relationship between itch, tingling and pain is obscure. The itch threshold varies according to the number of distractions, and most patients with a pruritic rash complain that the itch is worse at night.

The itch of different dermatoses is relieved by different types of scratching. Urticaria patients rarely have scratch marks, and scabies provokes only short excoriations. Atopic eczema patients often produce much larger scratches, with extensive bleeding, and patients with 'neurotic' excoriations (p. 191) gouge out chunks of skin. Eczematous patients often use the back of the nail plate to rub the irritable skin, and their nails become very highly polished.

GENERALIZED PRURITUS

Widespread itching with no apparent skin disease is a common complaint. Careful examination is needed to exclude scabies, lice, insect bites and dermatitis herpetiformis. Fibreglass dermatitis is another trap for the unwary. There may be no obvious history of loft insulating, boat-building etc; but Mum may have popped the fibreglass curtains in the washing machine with Dad's underpants.

Having excluded external cause so far as possible, appropriate examination and investigation is required to exclude the following systemic causes of pruritus:

1. *Hepatic disease.* Obstructive jaundice (especially biliary cirrhosis) causes pruritus, but the itch is due to bile salts, not bili-

rubin, and its severity therefore correlates poorly with the degree of jaundice. It is usually relieved by oral cholestyramine.

Generalized pruritus sometimes occurs in pregnancy or in women taking oral contraceptives, and this is due to oestrogen-induced cholestasis.

2. *Blood disease.* Myeloproliferative disorders, particularly polycythaemia vera, can cause severe intractable pruritus. Lymphoma too must be carefully excluded since the pruritus can present before obvious lymphadenopathy develops. Iron deficiency also causes pruritus, which is relieved by oral iron. In male patients, pruritus due to iron deficiency seems to be a marker for occult carcinoma of the gastro-intestinal tract.

3. *Carcinoma* of the internal organs may present with generalized pruritus, and this can precede detection of the neoplasm by several years.

4. *Chronic renal failure.* The cause of the severe itching in this disease is unknown. Some cases are due to secondary hyperparathyroidism and are relieved by parathyroidectomy. In other cases the dry skin is an important factor, and the itch responds to emollients. Dialysis seems to provoke the pruritus in some patients.

5. *Endocrine disease.* Pruritus is common in late pregnancy, sometimes with a non-specific urticated rash (p. 229).

Itching may occur in both hypo- and hyperthyroidism.

Many books mention diabetes mellitus as a cause of generalized itching, but this is in fact exceptionally rare (although pruritus vulvae is common).

6. *Drugs.* Cocaine and morphine cause itching in addicts by a pharmacological action, but a more important cause of pruritus is allergy to a drug such as penicillin or gold. In these cases the pruritus may precede the rash by days or even weeks.

7. *Parasites.* This is a rare cause in U.K., but onchocerciasis, trichinosis etc., can cause pruritus, usually with a marked eosinophilia.

In many cases of generalized pruritus, especially in elderly people, no cause can be found. The terms 'senile' pruritus and 'psychological' pruritus are sometimes used in such cases, but these terms should be avoided unless senility or psychological factors can be clearly implicated in the aetiology. Some patients with idiopathic generalized pruritus do have an overt personality defect, neurosis or psychosis, and the excoriations they produce are often so deep as to leave scars ('neurotic' excoriations).

Treatment of idiopathic pruritus

If the skin is dry the itching will often respond to emollients. Daily bathing should be discouraged, as this dries the skin and exacerbates the condition. Some cases will respond well to cholestyramine, cimetidine or UVB irradiation twice weekly. Other cases will require symptomatic treatment with antihistamines or sedatives, and chlorpromazine 25 mg t.d.s. is often useful in this situation. The patients must be reviewed periodically for the development of previously unrecognized disease.

LOCALIZED PRURITUS

1. Lichen simplex (localized 'neuro-dermatitis')

Lichenification is often secondary to eczema, but it can also occur in skin which previously appeared normal, and it is then called lichen simplex. It usually develops at a localized site such as the ankle or neck which is easy to reach, and can be scratched 'without thinking'. Itching occurs in paroxysms, and the scratching continues until the skin is sore, when relief is obtained until the next paroxysm occurs some hours later. If this 'itch-scratch' cycle can be broken the skin should completely clear. Intensive therapy with a steroid ointment under polythene occlusion is usually successful if the patient has the will-power to stop scratching for a week or two. It is important that localized contact dermatitis and tinea are excluded before this reassurance is given. Psychological tension appears to make lichen simplex worse, and a tranquillizer may be helpful. It should be remembered however that a certain amount of stress is an inescapable part of many competitive occupations and patients do not appreciate being sedated out of a job.

2. Nodular prurigo

In this uncommon but very troublesome disease, the patient develops scattered warty nodules, each about 1–2 cm in diameter, which are intensely itchy. The cause is unknown, but it sometimes develops as a complication of another pruritic dermatosis such as eczema, and it probably represents an idiosyncratic reaction to scratching. Histologically there is a gross accentuation of the changes found in lichenification together with a proliferation of nerve fibres in the dermis.

Infiltration of the nodules with triamcinolone usually relieves the itching.

3. Pruritus ani

Localized perianal itching is common in adult males and the following predisposing causes must be excluded

(i) Rectal or anal disease such as haemorrhoids or fissure-in-ano

(ii) Poor hygiene, diarrhoea or discharge causing soiling of the perianal skin

(iii) Contact dermatitis to toilet paper or local anaesthetic ointment

(iv) Localized dermatosis e.g., psoriasis, 'seborrhoeic' dermatitis, lichen planus, crab lice, tinea, erythrasma, Candidosis, peri-anal Paget's disease, etc.

(v) Threadworm infestation (especially in children).

Often no cause can be found, and psychoanalysts (with the accent on the psycho-anal) have stated that pruritus ani is a sign of latent homosexuality (presumably head-scratchers are even more perverse). Telling a patient that he is a latent homosexual is unlikely to enhance the doctor-patient relationship, and even if it is true, the knowledge is unlikely to lead to successful therapy of his pruritus ani.

Idiopathic pruritus ani may be treated by the regular application of the weakest steroid necessary to control the itching. In some cases with wrinkled perianal skin, the regular use of moist cotton wool instead of toilet paper may be helpful.

Pruritus vulvae

As with pruritus ani, many cases of pruritus vulvae are idiopathic and will require symptomatic treatment with steroid ointments, but there are also many organic causes, as follows:

(i) Vaginal discharge, especially due to Candidosis or trichomonas. Diabetes must be excluded in every patient with pruritus vulvae, even if there is no discharge.

(ii) Contact dermatitis due to contraceptives (rubber, spermicidal jelly, etc.) or deodorants

(iii) Threadworms

(iv) Localized dermatoses (see pruritus ani, above).

An important additional cause of pruritus vulvae is *lichen sclerosus et atrophicus* (Fig. 17.1). This chronic disease may be a variant of morphoea (p. 224) as the two conditions sometimes occur together. It is characterized by ivory-white atrophic areas around the vulva and anus and histology of these areas shows a band of hyalinized collagen beneath the epidermis. The condition occurs mainly in

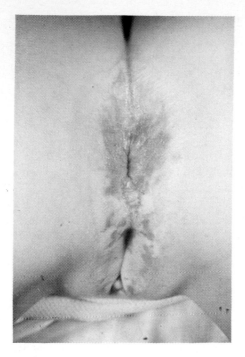

Fig. 17.1 Lichen sclerosus et atrophicus

middle-aged or elderly females. A similar condition occasionally affects the male foreskin (*balanitis xerotica*) though in this case it is often seen before puberty, as a cause of phimosis. Lichen sclerosus et atrophicus often progresses to leukoplakia, possibly as a result of prolonged scratching. Regular observation is necessary since leukoplakia is a premalignant condition, and suspect areas should be excised.

18

Blisters

A blister is a physical sign, not a disease, but because the differential diagnosis of a blistering eruption is a common clinical problem it is convenient to consider these heterogenous diseases together.

Mechanisms of blister formation

Blisters may be produced in a wide variety of ways, and they may form at various levels. In order to comprehend some recent advances in our understanding of blister formation, it is necessary to have some idea of the anatomy of the dermo-epidermal junction, as seen by electron microscopy.

The *dermo-epidermal junction* includes the basal cell layer, the basal lamina (which is electron-dense) and the upper papillary dermis (Fig. 18.1). The narrow space that separates the membrane of the basal cell from the basal lamina is called the lamina lucida. This

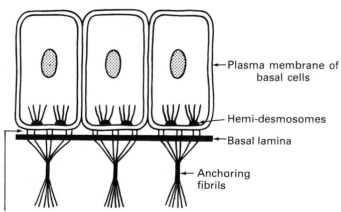

Fig. 18.1 The dermo-epidermal junction

195

space contains the bullous pemphigoid antigen (see p. 205), and a few anchoring filaments that cross from the basal cells to the basal lamina.

The following mechanisms occur:

1. Spongiosis

In eczema the keratinocytes become separated by the accumulation of oedema fluid (Fig. 18.2)

2. Epidermal cell necrosis

This occurs when the keratinocytes are invaded by a virus such as varicella or herpes simplex. The cells become swollen and vacuolated to produce an appearance called 'balloon degeneration'.

3. Damage to intercellular 'cement'

In pemphigus vulgaris, an auto-immune disease, antibodies directed against the intercellular cement cause the keratinocytes to lose

1. Spongiosis: inter-cellular oedema

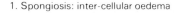

2. Balloon degeneration: cell death

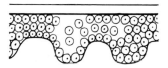

3. Acantholysis: loss of cell cohesion

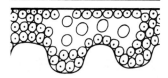

Fig. 18.2 Mechanisms for intra-epidermal blister formation

their cohesion and drift apart. This process is called acantholysis (the prickle cells of the Malpighian layer are acanthocytes) (Fig. 18.2).

4. Basal cell damage

Epidermolysis bullosa simplex (p. 206) causes disruption of the basal cells following mild trauma. Degeneration of the basal cell layer also occurs in lupus erythematosus and lichen planus, and on rare occasions this can be so severe as to produce bullae.

5. Damage to the lamina lucida

In bullous pemphigoid (p. 205) the split occurs at the level of the lamina lucida, presumably as a result of the IgG antibody binding with the bullous pemphigoid antigen at this site.

6. Dermal damage

(i) In recessive dystrophic epidermolysis bullosa (p. 206), the split occurs just below the basal lamina, and the anchoring fibrils are absent. In this condition there is increased collagenase activity.

(ii) In dermatitis herpetiformis (p. 201) there are granular deposits of IgA in the tips of the papillary dermis, and these are associated in the early stages with microabscesses due to neutrophil accumulation. It is thought that dapsone may exert its beneficial effect in this disease by inhibiting the neutrophil myeloperoxidase enzymes.

(iii) In porphyria cutanea tarda (p. 162) the blisters develop in the dermis, and there is considerable oedema of the dermal papillae, but relatively few inflammatory cells are found. Immunoglobulins and complement components accumulate around the dermal blood vessels, presumably as a result of damage caused by solar irradiation of the excess porphyrins in the blood.

Clinical classification of blistering eruptions

For clinical purposes, the bullous dermatoses are best classified according to the histological level of the split (Fig. 18.3):

Intra-epidermal	Sub-epidermal
1. Friction blisters	1. Burns
2. Eczema	2. Dermatitis herpetiformis
3. Infection	3. Erythema multiforme
4. Pemphigus vulgaris	4. Pemphigoid

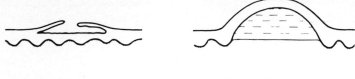

Intra-epidermal
blister ruptures easily

Sub epidermal
blister remains intact

Fig. 18.3 Classification of blisters

The two types can often be distinguished clinically, because the thin roof of the intra-epidermal blister easily ruptures, whereas the thicker roof of the sub-epidermal blister allows the formation of a tense, shiny, dome-shaped bulla. Blisters taken for biopsy must be fresh, because sub-epidermal blisters begin to re-epithelialize within 24 hours and they can then be mistaken for intra-epidermal blisters (Fig. 18.4).

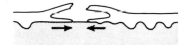

Fig. 18.4 Three day-old subepidermal blister showing re-epithelialization

A. INTRA-EPIDERMAL BLISTERS

1. Friction blisters

Despite much research funded by the U.S. Army (worried by the prevalence of blistered feet in Vietnam), we still do not fully understand the pathogenesis of friction blisters. One useful tip for self-medication is that sterile aspiration of a friction blister within 12 hr of its formation, followed by a pressure dressing, usually causes the roof to readhere, thus saving days of limping. The roof of a blister should not be removed, unless there is secondary infection.

2. Eczema

The blisters in eczema are usually small and multilocular. Large bullae, especially on the dorsum of the hands, should suggest the possibility of an exogenous cause.

3. Infection

(i) The regular grouped vesicles of herpes (simplex or zoster) are usually easy to diagnose.

(ii) Bullous impetigo is often misdiagnosed, especially in the early stages before the characteristic crusts have formed.

4. Pemphigus vulgaris

This is an uncommon chronic disease of unknown aetiology in which IgG antibody reacts with an antigen in the intercellular cement to cause intra-epidermal blisters (Fig. 18.5). The affected prickle cells become rounded, with clear cytoplasm, and they are then called acantholytic cells.

Pemphigus mainly affects middle-aged people, especially Jews, and if untreated it is eventually fatal. The onset is insidious, with widespread blisters which easily rupture to leave weeping tender erosions. *Nikolsky's sign* is usually present, i.e., if firm pressure is

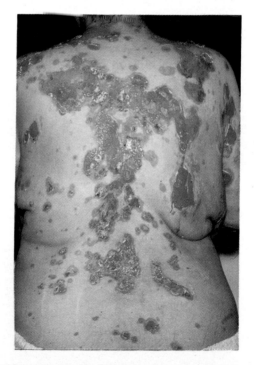

Fig. 18.5 Pemphigus vulgaris. The blisters rupture early in this disease

exerted on the 'normal' skin and a shearing strain is applied, a blister will be produced. The mucous membranes of the eyes, mouth, anus and genitalia are commonly involved.

Immunofluorescent testing

The diagnosis of pemphigus can be confirmed by biopsy of a fresh blister for histology and *direct immunofluorescent* testing. This is a technique in which antibody to human IgG is produced by injecting it into an animal. The animal's anti-human IgG antibody is then collected and labelled with a fluorescein marker. This labelled anti-human IgG is then incubated with the patient's skin, and if human IgG is attached to the intercellular cement, the animal anti-IgG antibody will recognize it, and after washing, the attached anti-IgG shows up as a pale green fluorescence in the epidermis (Fig. 18.6).

In practice, the pathologist uses several commercial antibodies directed against IgG, IgM, IgA and complement, so that the other auto-immune diseases can be excluded.

An alternative, but less reliable test, is the *indirect immunofluorescent* technique, in which the patient's serum is incubated with normal monkey oesophagus. If the pathological IgG is present in the serum it will become attached to the antigen present in the normal epithelial tissue, and it can be subsequently detected as above.

Treatment of pemphigus

Prednisone in high dosage (around 80 to 100 mg daily) is usually needed for a week or so to suppress the disease, and the dose can then be gradually reduced. The condition relapses if steroids are

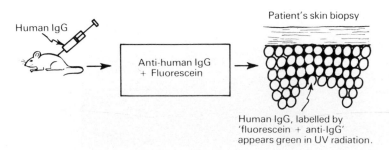

Fig. 18.6 Demonstration of intercellular IgG antibody in pemphigus vulgaris by immuno-fluorescent test

stopped, but the addition of azathioprine allows the steroid dose to be greatly reduced with relatively few side-effects.

B. SUB-EPIDERMAL BLISTERS

1. Burns

These are usually diagnosed from the history, but they can be easily misdiagnosed in hospital patients e.g., burns sustained during a general anaesthetic, or in patients with a sensory neuropathy. Syringomyelia patients for example are liable to sustain cigarette burns of the fingers.

2. Dermatitis herpetiformis

This is an uncommon chronic auto-immune disease in which IgA antibody is directed against an antigen in the dermo-epidermal junction.

It may begin at any age, and it usually starts with a nondescript itchy rash on the extensor surfaces of the knees, elbows or buttocks which resembles chronic eczema or urticaria (Fig 18.7). The irritation becomes severe, and eventually the rash begins to produce groups of small blisters.

It was discovered empirically that *dapsone* (normally used for leprosy) in a dose of about 100 mg daily causes dramatic resolution of the rash and the irritation.

This disease is of great academic interest because nearly every patient with dermatitis herpetiformis has a mild form of coeliac disease. The details of the relationship between oral gluten and cutaneous inflammation are obscure, but the primary pathology seems to be in the bowel. Dapsone therapy does not affect the malabsorption, but the introduction of a gluten-free diet causes a reduction in the dose of dapsone needed to suppress the rash. This is clinically helpful, since dapsone in high dosage often causes haemolysis.

3. Erythema multiforme

This is a distinctive eruption which is probably an immunological reaction to a variety of provocative factors such as infections (especially herpes simplex or mycoplasma) and drugs (especially long-acting sulphonamides). The hall-mark of the disease is the *target lesion* (Fig. 18.8), which has a pallid or purple centre surrounded

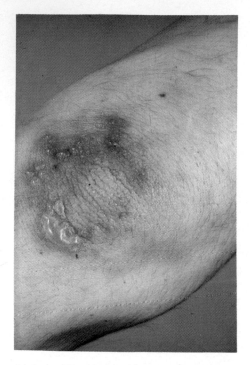

Fig. 18.7 Dermatitis herpetiformis of the elbow

by one or more red rings. This commonly occurs on the palmar surface of the hands. As the term multiforme implies, there may be a variety of other appearances ranging from red macules to large bullae (Fig. 18.9). The mucosa of the eyes, mouth and genitalia may be involved. The lesions come in crops and last for two or three weeks. Subsequent exposure to the initiating stimulus will cause a further attack.

The disease occurs in all degrees of severity and it can be fatal. The *Stevens-Johnson syndrome* (Fig. 18.10) is a severe form which may be associated with prostration, fever, pneumonitis and renal failure.

The skin histology shows severe inflammation at the epidermo-dermal junction, often with vasculitis in the dermis, but immuno-fluorescent tests are negative.

Treatment of erythema multiforme

Since the disease is self-limiting, mild cases require only sympto-

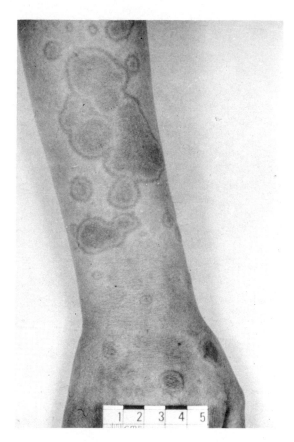

Fig. 18.8 Erythema multiforme, showing target lesions

matic treatment (e.g., mouth washes). Prednisone is usually prescribed for the more severe forms, though some trials have shown it is ineffective.

It is important to try to identify the causative antigen with a view to preventing subsequent attacks. Iodo-deoxyuridine should be used to treat herpes simplex, if this is present, in order to decrease the chance of recurrence.

Toxic epidermal necrolysis ('Scalded skin' syndrome)

This uncommon but potentially fatal disease may be a variant of erythema multiforme because the two conditions sometimes occur together. Clinically the skin becomes red, swollen and tender with

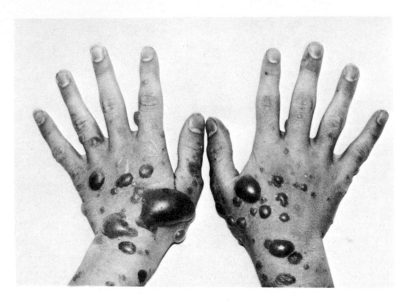

Fig. 18.9 Erythema multiforme, showing bullae

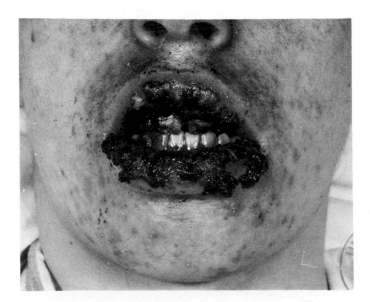

Fig. 18.10 Stevens-Johnson syndrome, showing the characteristic haemorrhagic crusting of the lips

desquamation of sheets of epidermis, so that it looks as though it had been scalded (Fig. 18.11). Histologically there is epidermal necrosis which may start at any level in the epidermis.

There are two types of toxic epidermal necrolysis. In adults, it is usually an immunological disease provoked by drug hypersensitivity, but in babies it is due to the direct necrolytic effect of a diffusible toxin produced by certain phage types of Staphylococci (p. 128).

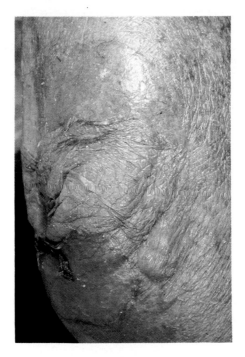

Fig. 18.11 Toxic epidermal necrolysis

4. Pemphigoid

This is an uncommon auto-immune disease of the elderly. In the classical form there are widespread large tense bullae which develop on areas of urticated erythema (Fig. 18.12).

Sometimes the disease resembles pemphigus, but mucosal involvement is unusual in pemphigoid. Histology of a fresh blister will show a sub-epidermal split, and immunofluorescent testing shows IgG directed against the specific antigen in the lamina lucida of the dermo-epidermal junction.

Treatment

This is the same as for pemphigus, but lower doses of steroids are required and pemphigoid pursues a more benign course, being likely to go into remission within a few years of onset.

5. Epidermolysis bullosa

Epidermolysis bullosa is a group of at least five genetic diseases, which vary in their severity, inheritance and pathogenesis. In the commonest type (epidermolysis bullosa simplex) which is due to a dominant gene, blisters occur only on the palms and soles following mild trauma, particularly in hot weather. In the rarer but more severe types such as recessive dystrophic epidermolysis bullosa, there may be such widespread blistering and scarring of the skin and mucosal surfaces that death occurs 'in utero' or soon after delivery.

6. Other diseases which cause blisters

(i)   Drugs e.g., nalidixic acid and barbiturate overdose
(ii) Insect bites (p. 146)
(iii) Porphyria (p. 162)
(iv) Vasculitis (p. 171)

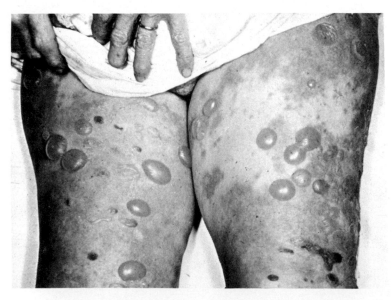

Fig. 18.12 Bullous pemphigoid, showing dome-shaped blisters arising on areas of erythema

19

Immunopathology and the skin

Immunological reactions play a major part in the pathogenesis of many skin diseases. Sometimes these are normal reactions which constitute part of the body's defence against a pathogen (e.g., granuloma formation in lupus vulgaris) and sometimes they are aberrant reactions (e.g., auto-immune disease such as pemphigoid). Several distinct types of allergic reaction are recognized, and these are useful concepts, but it is important to realize that not all immunological diseases fit neatly into one or other type, and there is often considerable overlap, with several reactions proceeding simultaneously or consecutively. Inflammation may also be produced by nonimmune mechanisms e.g., some spider venoms can activate complement directly.

The *Langerhans cell* which is found in the epidermis (p. 9) is now considered part of the immune system. Routine histology of the Langerhans cells shows a resemblance to the melanocyte, but electron microscopy shows marked differences and Langerhans cells contain characteristic racquet-shaped bodies in their cytoplasm. Langerhans cells are probably modified macrophages which originate in the marrow and then move to the epidermis. They can 'recognize' antigens reaching the skin surface and transfer this information to the dermal lymphocytes. They are thus the most peripheral part of the afferent limb of the immune system. The rare disease 'histiocytosis X' is due to abnormal proliferation of Langerhans cells.

CLASSIFICATION OF HARMFUL ALLERGIC REACTIONS

Type 1. Anaphylactic ('immediate hypersensitivity') (Fig. 19.1)

In this reaction, a circulating IgE antibody (reaginic antibody) becomes bound to tissue cells such as the mast cell. When the antigen, which is often a foreign protein (e.g., pollen or food), comes into contact with two adjacent antibody molecules it causes the mast cell

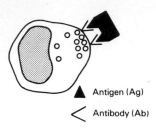

Antigen (Ag)

Antibody (Ab)

granules to be attracted to the surface of the cell, and histamine and other vasoactive substances are then discharged from the granules to the exterior. Eosinophils are attracted to the site of the reaction, but their role is not yet clear.

Anaphylaxis, in which there is massive histamine release throughout the body, is the classical example of this type of reaction. Hay-fever and some types of asthma and urticaria are also good examples.

A substance suspected of causing a Type 1 reaction can be tested *in vivo* by inoculating it into the forearm skin by a small scratch. This is called a *prick test*. A positive reaction produces a white weal on an erythematous base, often with 'pseudopodia'. This develops within 20 minutes and resolves within 2 hr. Control inoculations are essential. A battery of common pollens and mould can be quickly tested to identify the allergen in patients with hay-fever, prior to a course of desensitizing infections.

Type 2. Cytotoxic (Fig. 19.2)

In this reaction the antibody, which is usually IgG or IgM, reacts with an antigen which is bound to a cell surface. The reaction usually involves complement activation, and eventual damage to the affected cells. Red blood cells are classically involved in this type of reaction (e.g., haemolysis in transfusion reactions), but auto-immune skin diseases such as pemphigus, pemphigoid, dermatitis herpetiformis and lupus erythematosus may also involve Type 2 reactions.

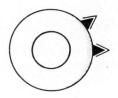

There is no suitable *in vivo* test for Type 2 reactions, but skin biopsy and immunofluorescent testing allows antibody fixed to cells or cell products (e.g., basement membranes) to be identified.

Type 3. Arthus ('Circulating immune-complexes') (Fig. 19.3)

This reaction occurs when antigen and antibody are both present in the circulation in roughly equi-molar proportions. The resulting 'immune-complexes' tend to precipitate in small blood vessels, initiating complement activation and an intense inflammatory reaction. Recent work suggests that circulating immune-complexes do not always cause tissue damage, but they probably play an important role in the pathogenesis of glomerulonephritis, arthritis and vasculitis in many 'immunological' diseases.

'Serum sickness' is the classical example of this reaction, but this should not occur now that we no longer inject people with foreign proteins such as horse-serum. Dermatologists see many diseases in which immune-complexes are involved, e.g., lupus erythematosus, polyarteritis nodosa, Henoch-Schönlein purpura, erythema nodosum, etc. Sometimes a bacterial, viral or drug antigen can be identified, but in many cases the allergen is obscure.

Increasingly sophisticated immunological techniques are now being used to try to identify the antigen in immune complexes. Clinically a Type 3 reaction can be identified by injecting the suspected antigen intradermally. A positive reaction produces an ill-defined red swelling, sometimes purpuric, which develops over several hours and resolves in 24–36 hr.

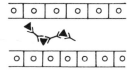

Type 4. Cell-mediated ('delayed hypersensitivity') (Fig. 19.4)

In this reaction, sensitized lymphocytes react with antigen deposited at a local site to provoke a complicated, slowly evolving, mixed cellular reaction which involves T cells, B cells and macrophages. During this reaction the sensitized lymphocytes release ill-defined substances called *lymphokines*, which recruit non-sensitized lymphocytes to the area and amplify the immune response. The best-known lymphokine is the '*macrophage migration inhibition factor*'

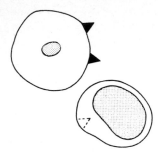

(MIF) which appears to cause macrophage aggregation. Another important lymphokine is the *mitogenic factor* which induces lymphocyte proliferation.

The 'tuberculin reaction' is the classical Type 4 reaction, but contact dermatitis is another good example. This type of hypersensitivity can be demonstrated *in vivo* either by intra-dermal injection or by a *patch test*. A positive reaction consists of an indurated red area, sometimes with vesiculation, which develops over 24–48 hr and resolves over several days. Simple molecules such as nickel are not themselves antigenic, but they act as *haptens* and become antigenic by combining with proteins in the skin.

Some chemicals such as dinitro-chlorobenzene (DNCB) are such potent sensitizers that virtually all normal subjects readily develop delayed hypersensitivity to them. DNCB applied in serial patch tests can thus be used to test the competence of the immune response e.g., in patients with malignancy or recurrent infections.

Type 5. Antibody-dependent cell-mediated cytotoxicity

This is a mixed form in which two types of non-immune killer cells (K cells) act in conjunction with antibody to damage target cells. These mixed reactions may be important in certain auto-immune diseases, and in immunological reactions to malignancy (e.g., melanoma).

Type 6. Granuloma formation

Granulomata arise as an inflammatory response to a wide variety of infective agents and irritant substances. Allergic reactions (particularly allergic vasculitis and Type 4 reactions) are sometimes associated with granuloma formation. Granulomatous skin diseases include tuberculosis, leprosy, syphilis, sarcoidosis, granuloma annulare and necrobiosis lipoidica.

Possible 'immunological' diseases

In addition to the disorders mentioned above there are several diseases of unknown aetiology in the pathogenesis of which immune reactions appear to play a part. It may be that future work will reveal a specific mechanism which will enable them to be classified more rationally, but for the present it is convenient to consider them in this chapter as an unrelated miscellany.

Lichen planus

This chronic disease is characterized by extremely itchy, shiny, flat-topped, pinkish-purple papules which eventually resolve to leave pigmented macules. Close inspection of their surface reveals a network of thin white lines (Wickham's striae).

The eruption usually starts suddenly on the flexor aspect of the wrists (Fig. 19.5) and then spreads to the trunk and shins, and in the latter site the papules tend to coalesce into a hypertrophic plaque (Fig. 19.6). The palms and soles may be involved, and there may be a variety of nail changes, ranging from pits or ridges to complete loss of the nail.

Mouth lesions are an important aid to diagnosis, though they do not occur in every case. A white lacy network on the buccal mucosa opposite the pre-molars (Fig. 19.7) is the usual pattern, but the lips and tongue may also be involved. In severe cases there is marked

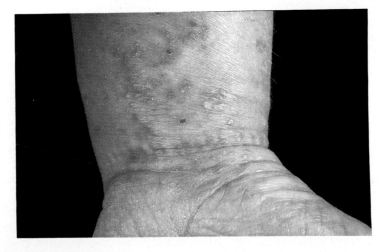

Fig. 19.5 Lichen planus

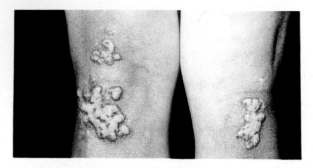

Fig. 19.6 Lichen planus of the hypertrophic type

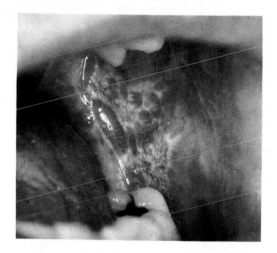

Fig. 19.7 Lichen planus of the oral mucosa

inflammation and even ulceration. These severe changes are pre-malignant and should be reviewed periodically.

The histology of lichen planus is striking (Fig. 19.8) A dense band-like infiltrate of lymphocytes 'hugs' the lower surface of the epidermis. The epidermis itself becomes thickened, its lower border assumes a 'saw-tooth' pattern, and the basal layer undergoes patchy degeneration. A variety of changes have been reported on immuno-fluorescent testing.

These changes, together with the response to steroid therapy, suggest an immunological involvement. This idea is supported by that the 'graft-versus-host' reaction following bone-marrow trans-plants can provoke the onset of lichen planus. A wide variety of

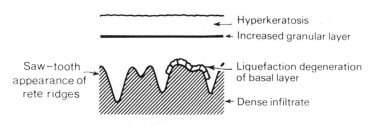

Fig. 19.8 Histology of lichen planus

drugs, including gold, amiphenazole and anti-malarials, can also provoke a rash which is virtually indistinguishable from lichen planus.

Treatment

The course is variable, with new lesions appearing at regular intervals, but many cases clear within a year. There is no specific cure, but resolution seems to be helped by topical steroids. Polythene occlusion and even systemic steroids may be needed in severe cases. Chronic hypertrophic lesions can be injected with triamcinolone.

If oral lesions are painful they should be treated with triamcinolone in Orabase, applied q.d.s.

Pyoderma gangrenosum

This is a chronic inflammatory process which produces an irregular ulcer with an overhanging purple edge and a necrotic base (Fig. 19.9). The lesions may begin as a pustule or a tender nodule, but this are sterile on bacteriological culture. The lesions may occur singly or in crops.

Many predisposing causes have been identified, including ulcerative colitis, rheumatoid disease, dysproteinaemia etc. but the pathogenesis remains a mystery.

The treatment is unsatisfactory if no underlying cause can be found and treated. Injection of triamcinolone beneath the ulcer may help, and in more severe cases, systemic steroids, cytotoxic drugs or dapsone may be tried.

Aphthae (aphthous ulcers)

These small mouth ulcers develop at some time or another in at

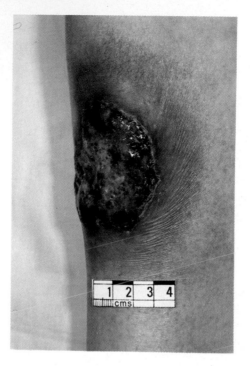

Fig. 19.9 Pyoderma gangrenosum

least 20 per cent of the population, and yet their cause is obscure. An auto-immune disorder is one fashionable hypothesis. They start as small red macules on the buccal mucosa which rapidly erode to form a painful shallow ulcer with a yellow base. They heal spontaneously in about a week, but recurrence at more or less regular intervals is common. In some cases the recurrences appear to be provoked by stress or by trauma such as vigorous tooth-brushing.

As might be expected for such a common and mysterious disease, treatments are legion, but no cure is known. Recommended therapy includes tetracycline suspension (250 mg in 5 ml) mouth washes, triamcinolone in Orabase, and freezing with liquid nitrogen.

It should be mentioned in passing that many general practitioners fail to recognize malignant ulcers in the mouth, and label them as aphthous ulcers. A mouth ulcer which persists for more than 3 weeks should be biopsied unless the cause is clearly identified.

Behcet's syndrome is a rare disease in which large ulcers resembling aphthae occur in the mouth and around the genitalia. There may also be widespread sterile pustules, conjunctivitis and uveitis, thrombophlebitis and widespread necrotic foci in the central nervous system.

Reiter's disease

This uncommon syndrome mainly affects young men. It is precipitated either by non-specific urethritis or dysentery. About two weeks after the initial urethritis or enteritis the patient develops conjunctivitis or uveitis, arthritis, balanitis and stomatitis. There may be a red hyperkeratotic rash on the soles called 'keratoderma blenorrhagica' which is sometimes indistinguishable from pustular psoriasis.

The pathogenesis of this disease is obscure, but it is presumed to be an immunological reaction to the original infective agent.

Sarcoidosis

This is another intriguing disease which is hard to define. It is characterized by the presence in several organs of epithelioid cell tubercles without caseation, though some fibrinoid necrosis may be present. This is the histological appearance of a foreign-body granuloma, and it seems that patients with sarcoidosis readily produce granulomata throughout the body in response to unidentified stimuli.

The commonest change is a bilateral hilar lymphadenopathy which is often asymptomatic. This is followed by a pulmonary infiltrate which either resolves or progresses to fibrosis. Many other organs may be involved, particularly the liver, spleen, eyes, bones, nervous system and skin.

There are many patterns of skin involvement but granulomata in the skin are often recognizable as firm dermal nodules with a shiny, rather translucent, appearance. A biopsy is almost always needed, and a Kveim test may be required if no evidence of sarcoidosis in other organs can be detected.

'Lupus pernio' is a distinctive form in which soft bluish-red plaques resembling chilblains occur on the nose, cheeks and ears (Fig. 19.10). The tendency of sarcoidosis to arise in cutaneous scars is probably due to the presence of microscopic foreign bodies in the scar.

Erythema nodosum may be a common feature of sarcoidosis, but it is due to circulating immune complexes and is not a granulomatous reaction.

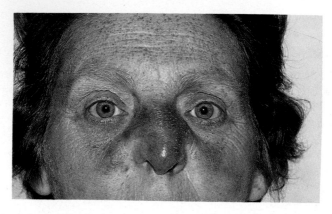

Fig. 19.10 Sarcoidosis of the lupus pernio type. The nasal bones are also affected by cysts due to sarcoid

Treatment of sarcoidosis

The decision as to whether systemic steroids should be given for sarcoidosis of internal organs is often difficult, since the disease eventually remits spontaneously. Indications for steroid therapy include uveitis, breathlessness, hypercalcaemia and myocardial or neurological involvement. In most forms of cutaneous sarcoidosis, intra-lesional injection of triamcinolone is preferable to systemic steroid therapy. Methotrexate has given good results in some severe cases.

20

The skin and systemic disease

CUTANEOUS EFFECTS OF SYSTEMIC DISEASE

Dermatology is a subject of peculiar charms (apart from those used for warts), and one of these is the frequency with which unsuspected internal disease is discovered by examination of the skin. Some dermatologists even claim to be the last of the general physicians! Several examples of skin changes due to underlying disease have been mentioned in previous chapters, but the following conditions are worth special attention.

A. COLLAGEN — VASCULAR DISEASE

1. Lupus erythematosus

Lupus erythematosus (LE) is an auto-immune disease which occurs in two main forms, *discoid* (DLE) which is confined to the skin, and *systemic* (SLE) which also affects the internal organs. The rash is different in the two types and there is some debate as to whether they are separate diseases, although they sometimes share serological abnormalities, and about 5 per cent of patients with DLE eventually develop SLE.

a. Discoid lupus (DLE)

This is a distinctive patchy rash which usually affects the face and neck and is exacerbated by sunlight. It consists of well-defined erythematous plaques, often with some degree of scaling, atrophy and follicular plugging (Fig. 20.1). When the scale is detached the keratin plugs can often be seen on the undersurface of the scale, giving a so-called 'carpet-tack' appearance (Fig. 20.2). Loss of pigment is common and in the later stages there is scarring. The scalp may be affected, with patches of scarring alopecia, and there may be crusting and erosions of the lips.

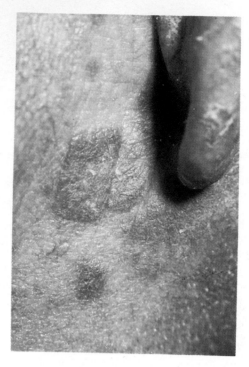

Fig. 20.1 Discoid lupus erythematosus

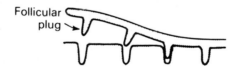

Fig. 20.2 'Carpet-tack' scale of discoid LE

The diagnosis is confirmed by biopsy of the involved skin. The histology shows hyperkeratosis, follicular plugs, 'liquefaction-degeneration' of the epidermal basal layer and dermal oedema with a patchy lymphocytic infiltrate. Immuno-fluorescent testing reveals that IgG or IgM are deposited in the basement membrane zone. About 20 per cent of cases have other laboratory abnormalities such as mild anaemia or leucopenia, hypergamma-globulinaemia, positive rheumatoid or anti-nuclear factor, etc. The DNA-antibody titre is usually low, even if ANF is present.

Treatment of DLE

DLE is a chronic disfiguring disease, but much can be done to mitigate the damage. Topical steroids are helpful, and this is one of the few diseases in which the more potent preparations may be used on the face. Sunlight must be avoided as far as possible, and topical sunscreens are advisable in the summer. In the more severe cases, antimalarial drugs such as hydroxychloroquine will suppress the disease but the long-term use of this drug is limited by the risk of retinal damage. Cosmetic covering creams often produce a dramatic improvement, especially for depigmented scars.

b. Systemic lupus (SLE)

This is a multisystem disease characterized by a tendency to pancytopenia and immunological abnormalities, especially antibodies to nuclear antigens. It usually presents in females aged 20 to 50, and the clinical features are as follows:

  (i) Fever, malaise or weight loss
 (ii) Arthralgia, often flitting or episodic
(iii) Skin changes or Raynaud's phenomenon (see below)
(iv) Renal involvement (glomerulonephritis,nephrotic syndrome or hypertension)
  (v) Pleurisy with effusion, or pneumonitis
 (vi) Lymphadenopathy
(vii) Myocarditis, endocarditis or pericarditis
(viii) Psychosis or neurological lesions, including epilepsy
 (ix) Hepatomegaly and splenomegaly

The prognosis is variable, but death can occur from malignant hypertension secondary to glomerulonephritis, or from neurological damage. Laboratory tests provide a notoriously poor guide to the disease activity, especially in the brain.

The rash of SLE is a symmetrical, blotchy erythema which characteristically involves the nose and malar regions ('butterfly rash') (Fig. 20.3) but any light-exposed area may be affected. Occasionally the rash is urticated or even purpuric. Diffuse alopecia is common, and provides a useful sign for monitoring disease activity.

Particular attention must be given to the hands in cases of suspected SLE. There may be erythema of the thenar or hypothenar areas. The fingers may be red, or there may be chilblain-like

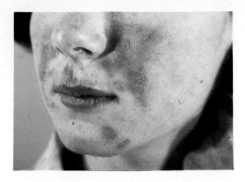

Fig. 20.3 Systemic lupus erythematosus ('butterfly' rash)

plaques. The nail-fold capillaries may be seen through a lens to be irregularly dilated (Fig. 20.4) and there may be splinter haemorrhages or small periungual infarcts due to vasculitis. There may be a history of Raynaud's phenomenon, but this is usually mild.

Diagnosis of SLE

The best single diagnostic criterion for SLE is a high titre of antibody to purified double-stranded DNA. Even if multiple criteria are used, however, some borderline cases are found to overlap with other collagen-vascular diseases such as rheumatoid disease.

The borderline between DLE and SLE is also similarly blurred on occasion, but in SLE there are usually marked haematological and serological abnormalities, with a high titre of DNA antibodies. A skin biopsy taken from apparently normal skin in a light-exposed area (e.g., the wrist) will often show positive immunofluorescence in SLE.

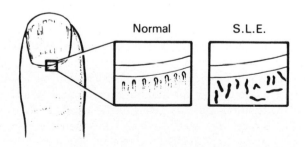

Fig. 20.4 Dilated nail-fold capillaries of systemic LE

Aetiology of SLE

Certain strains of NZB mice have a strong inherited predisposition to SLE and there is some evidence that humans also have a genetic predisposition to the disease. The 'trigger factor' is usually unknown, but recent work suggests that C-type viruses may be involved in the pathogenesis of some cases of SLE. Some drugs, especially hydrallazine and procainamide, can also provoke an SLE-like syndrome.

Treatment

The prognosis of SLE is variable, but severe vasculitis and renal or CNS involvement are ill omens. Systemic steroids form the mainstay of treatment but immunosuppressive drugs and antimalarials are also used. Plasmapheresis, which 'washes' immune-complexes from the blood has also been used successfully for severe cases.

2. Dermatomyositis

This is an uncommon disease in which cutaneous erythema and oedema is associated with an inflammatory myopathy. In the adult, about 25 to 50 per cent of cases are associated with an underlying carcinoma, but dermatomyositis which starts in childhood does not have this sinister connotation.

The rash is often an ill-defined erythema, but violaceous discoloration of the upper eyelids, red scaly patches over the knuckles, and ragged cuticles with nailfold capillary dilatation are distinctive features (Fig. 20.5). The histology often resembles lupus erythematosus but tests for immunofluorescence are negative. The myopathy tends to be proximal, and tests of muscle power should include asking the patient to sit up from the supine position without using the arms. Electromyography, serum enzyme measurements (aldolase, creatine kinase and amino-transferase) and biopsy of an affected muscle may help to confirm the diagnosis.

Treatment of dermatomyositis

Cases which are secondary to internal carcinoma may remit when the tumour is excised. In other cases prednisone or immunosuppressive drugs may be needed to relieve the myopathy, which may be life-threatening if the respiratory muscles are involved. In the

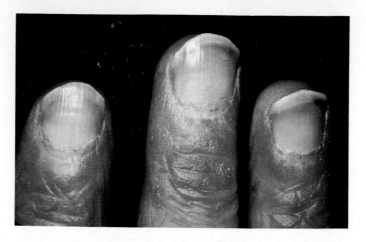

Fig. 20.5 Dermatomyositis, showing the characteristic rash over the knuckles, the irregular cuticles and the small nail-fold haemorrhages

juvenile form the prognosis for life is good, but deformity due to muscle fibrosis and contractures is common unless the disease can be suppressed.

3. Systemic sclerosis

This is a mysterious disease of unknown aetiology, which is characterized by excessive collagen deposition and arterial constriction and occlusion in several organs, particularly the skin, lungs, gastro-intestinal tract and kidneys.

Raynaud's phenomenon is the usual presenting symptom, and after some months or years the digital ischaemia becomes more severe, with finger-tip ulceration, loss of print pattern and eventual gangrene. The skin of the hands and face becomes progressively indurated and 'bound down' to the underlying tissue (Fig. 20.6). Facial movements become restricted, and the mouth becomes smaller. with radial furrows which give the appearance of premature ageing (Fig. 20.7). Loss of soft tissue from the nose produces a resemblance to a beak. Telangiectasia may develop on the cheeks. The facial appearance in a typical case is therefore pathognomonic, and patients with this disease often look like siblings. Less common cutaneous changes include pigmentation and calcinosis (calcium deposition).

Pulmonary fibrosis develops in most patients, with exertional dyspnoea. Loss of peristalsis is also common, with consequent

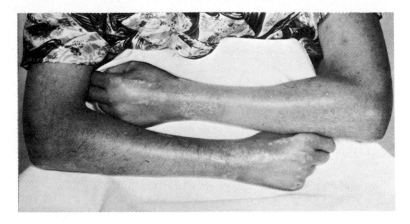

Fig. 20.6 Systemic sclerosis, showing the shiny indurated skin

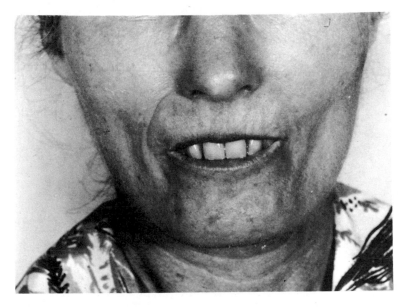

Fig. 20.7 Systemic sclerosis, showing the 'tight' mouth, with perioral wrinkles

'heartburn' or dysphagia. Colicky pain, distension and disturbance of bowel habit may occur due to intestinal involvement. Renal failure or malignant hypertension is a common terminal event in these patients, and it may develop with dramatic rapidity.

Laboratory confirmation of the diagnosis is often difficult to obtain. There may be a variety of serological abnormalities, including positive tests for rheumatoid factor, ANF, etc. Skin biopsy is rarely helpful in doubtful cases.

Treatment of systemic sclerosis

Steroids and immunosuppressive drugs are notoriously disappointing in this disease. Penicillamine, which prevents the stabilization of new collagen, will help the skin sclerosis, but has little effect on the more serious systemic changes. Recent work suggests that powerful vasodilators such as minoxidil may be helpful. Prostacyclin infusion or oral nifedipine may help the digital ischaemia.

Morphoea

This is an idiopathic disorder in which there is localized sclerosis of the skin. It usually presents with a large oval plaque of a violaceous hue (Fig. 20.8) which gradually becomes indurated and assumes an ivory colour. The surface often appears smooth and shiny, with a decrease in sweat production, and loss of hairs. Usually no treatment is necessary, but in the rare generalized form the tightly-bound inelastic skin may hamper respiration and in these cases, penicillamine may be helpful.

The relationship between morphoea and systemic sclerosis is controversial, since morphoea occasionally precedes the development of systemic sclerosis, but unlike discoid LE, serological abnormalities do not occur in localized morphoea.

4. Mixed connective tissue disease

This condition usually presents with severe Raynaud's disease, and though it may have features of SLE, dermatomyositis and systemic sclerosis, the prognosis is relatively good. The diagnosis is confirmed by finding a circulating antibody to a specific ribonucleoprotein ('extractable nuclear antigen'), which is not found in systemic sclerosis. The DNA antibody titre in mixed connective tissue disease is normal.

5. Rheumatoid disease

The common dermatological manifestations of rheumatoid disease are as follows:

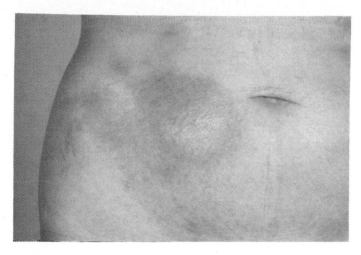

Fig. 20.8 Morphoea

(i) *Thin skin*

Patients with rheumatoid disease tend to have thin skin due to loss of collagen. Systemic steroid therapy aggravates this, and leads to easy bruising.

(ii) *Rheumatoid nodules*

These are firm subcutaneous nodules which commonly occur on the ulnar border of the forearm. They are usually associated with more severe forms of the disease, and they tend to ulcerate with trauma. Their histology is virtually identical to that of granuloma annulare.

(iii) *Vasculitis*

Digital vasculitis often causes small brown infarcts around the nails. Occasionally the skin elsewhere shows purpura or necrosis due to vasculitis, and rarely there may be gangrene of the hand or foot.

(iv) *Pressure sores*

(v) *Leg ulcers*

These occur more commonly in rheumatoid disease, and the predisposing factors include anaemia, thin skin, immobility, vasculitis and sensory neuropathy.

(vi) *Pyoderma gangrenosum (p. 213).*

Still's disease (Juvenile chronic polyarthritis)

About 25 per cent of patients with Still's disease have a transient rash, which consists of small pink maculo-papules with an irregular margin. The lesions do not expand and this distinguishes the rash from that of rheumatic fever.

6. Rheumatic fever

The characteristic rash is *erythema marginatum*, which appears as evanescent, pink rings on the trunk, which disappear without trace in a few hours but recur in crops. Less commonly, there may be urticaria, petechiae, nodules or erythema multiforme.

B. METABOLIC, ENDOCRINE AND NUTRITIONAL DISEASE

The cutaneous complications of these diseases are as follows:

1. Diabetes mellitus

(i) *Cutaneous infections* are common. Diabetics have an increased susceptibility to staphylococcal infection and Candidosis, and boils or pruritus vulvae may be the first sign of diabetes.

(ii) *Vascular occlusion* commonly causes gangrene of the toes or perforating ulcers of the soles. Diabetic neuropathy also predisposes to ulceration. Diabetic patients must pay particular attention to their footwear, and elderly diabetics should visit a chiropodist regularly.

(iii) *Brown scars* over the shins are common. They are apparently not due to trauma and for lack of information regarding aetiology they are simply called 'diabetic dermopathy'.

(iv) *Hyperlipidaemia* is a feature of uncontrolled diabetes and secondary xanthomata may appear as a crop of pink papules, especially over the buttocks (p. 229).

(v) *Necrobiosis lipoidica* is a rare disease but more than half the affected patients are diabetic. It appears as a reddish-brown patch, which slowly enlarges and becomes yellowish and atrophic, so that vessels can be seen through the shiny skin (Fig. 20.9). The shins and forehead are the usual sites. Histologically the lesions show collagen degeneration surrounded by epithelioid cells and giant cells.

(vi) *Granuloma annulare* produces firm skin-coloured papules which tend to be grouped in a ring on the back of the hand (Fig. 20.10). If the papules are painful or disfiguring they can be

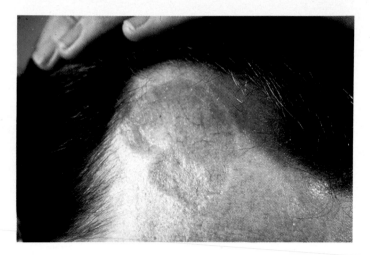

Fig. 20.9 Necrobiosis lipoidica

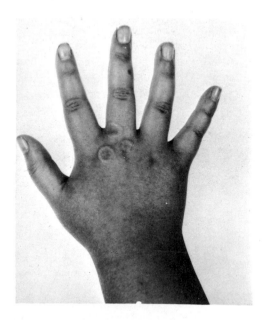

Fig. 20.10 Granuloma annulare

treated with intra-dermal injections of triamcinolone. The histology is almost identical with that of necrobiosis lipoidica and rheumatoid nodule.

Very few patients with localized granuloma annulare are diabetic, but there is a much rarer generalized form of the disease in which the incidence of diabetes is high.

(vii) *Insulin injections* may cause a variety of problems, including hypertrophy or atrophy at the injected site, and widespread urticaria due to impurities.

(viii) *Flushing* develops after alcohol ingestion in some patients receiving chlorpropamide therapy. This can be blocked by naloxone, which is an opiate antagonist, and mimicked by an enkephalin analogue with opiate activity, suggesting that endogenous opiates are responsible for the reaction. The opioids affect carbohydrate metabolism and insulin release, and it has been suggested that endogenous opioids may have a role in the pathogenesis of diabetes mellitus.

2. Hypothyroidism

In severe hypothyroidism the cold, dry, pale, puffy skin with thin hair and sparse eyebrows is pathognomonic. Often the skin has a yellowish tinge due to increased carotene. Elderly patients sometimes present with 'erythema ab igne' of the legs due to prolonged huddling over a fire. The word 'myxoedema' refers to connective tissue oedema due to mucin deposition.

3. Hyperthyroidism

The skin is often pink, soft, smooth and moist, and patients sometimes present with generalized hyperhidrosis. There may be diffuse alopecia with fine hair. Pigmentation may be increased, and there may be clubbing or onycholysis.

Pre-tibial myxoedema

Patients with hyperthyroidism associated with 'long-acting thyroid stimulator' (LATS) sometimes develop symmetrical plaques of mucinous oedema over the front of the shins. Potent steroid ointments applied to the affected area under polythene occlusion each night will diminish the lesions.

4. Acromegaly

The skin and subcutaneous tissues become hypertrophic and thickened, and both sweat and sebaceous glands are overactive so that the skin is moist and greasy. Increased pigmentation may occur, and skin tags are common.

5. Cushing's disease

In this disease the subcutaneous fat is redistributed, so that the trunk becomes obese, with a 'buffalo hump', while the limbs remain slim. The plethoric 'moon face' (Cushingoid facies) is pathognomonic of increased circulating gluco-corticoids. Thinning of the skin due to collagen loss may result in large purple striae. Cushing's disease increases susceptibility to cutaneous infections, especially Candidosis and pityriasis versicolor.

If adrenal androgens are also produced in excess there may be hirsutism, seborrhoea and acne.

6. Pregnancy

This is a self limiting disorder in which metabolic and endocrine derangements reach heroinic proportions. The common cutaneous events include striae ('stretch-marks') of the breasts and abdomen, increased pigmentation, and in the post-partum period, hair loss (p. 36). Spider naevi and palmar erythema are common, 'moles' tend to enlarge, and genital warts and Candidosis get worse, but the effect on most other skin diseases tends to be unpredictable.

Pruritus and various non-specific rashes are not uncommon in late pregnancy.

Pemphigoid gestationis (formerly called herpes gestationis) is a rare blistering disease of pregnancy which recurs in successive pregnancies. Immunofluorescent skin tests suggest that this is a form of bullous pemphigoid. It probably develops as an immunological reaction to the products of conception. The babies tend to be 'small for dates', and the incidence of still births is increased.

7. Xanthomata

A xanthoma is a collection of lipid-filled histiocytic cells in the skin. Xanthomata are usually (but not always) the result of increased plasma lipids, and this *hyperlipidaemia* may itself be *primary* (due to a genetic defect in fat metabolism) or *secondary* to acquired metabolic disease such as biliary tract obstruction, diabetes mellitus, myxoedema or the nephrotic syndrome.

Xanthomata may present a variety of appearances. Yellowish plaques around the eyelids (xanthelasma) are the commonest lesions, and about 50 per cent of such patients have hypercholesterolaemia with a tendency to atheroma and a family history of premature vascular occlusion. Other xanthomata may appear as firm yellow nodules (often on the knees and elbows) (Fig. 20.11), linear yellow deposits in the palms, lumps in the extensor tendons, large flat plaques (often on the forehead) or crops of small red-brown papules (often on the buttocks).

The treatment of xanthomata requires specialist advice. There are at least five biochemical types of hyperlipidemia, and the treatment of xanthomata depends upon the particular pattern of chylomicrons, triglycerides and lipoproteins found on laboratory testing. Most cases require dietary restrictions and drugs such as clofibrate (Atromid-S). If all laboratory tests are normal, xanthelasmata may be rendered less conspicuous by the careful application of trichloracetic acid.

8. Acrodermatitis enteropathica

This is a rare disease of young children which may be fatal if untreated. The basic defect is a decreased ability to absorb dietary zinc. The onset is insidious, with failure to thrive, a red scaly rash (often mistaken for psoriasis or Candidosis), hair loss and diarrhoea. Plasma zinc levels are low, but replacement therapy with high doses of oral zinc produces clinical improvement.

9. Scurvy

Though vitamin C is readily available in Britain, sporadic cases of scurvy are still seen occasionally in the elderly, in alcoholics and in those with food fads. The classical signs of scurvy include perifollicular purpura, swollen bleeding gums and poor wound healing, but an important presentation in the elderly is a brown, indurated oedema of the lower legs.

10. Pellagra

This is a systemic disease caused by nicotinic acid deficiency, which classically causes the 3D triad — 'dermatitis, diarrhoea and dementia'. The red scaly rash starts in light-exposed areas, and its clearly defined edge on the neck often produces a 'necklace' effect.

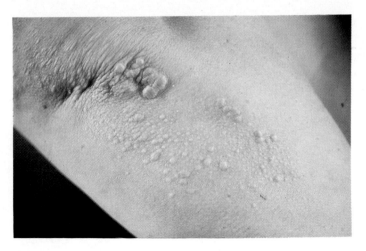

Fig. 20.11 Xanthomata due to hyperlipidaemia

11. Kwashiorkor

In conditions of famine, chronic deficiency of protein and vitamins in early life produces a complex syndrome with retardation of mental and skeletal development, muscle wasting and oedema. The skin becomes red and flaky and the hair of Negroes becomes a light reddish-brown. Mucosal lesions of the mouth, eyes and vulva are common.

Many other vitamins and trace elements (vitamin A, essential fatty acids, etc.) are important for cutaneous health but such deficiencies rarely occur in isolation.

Other skin changes secondary to systemic metabolic or endocrine disease include cutaneous virilization (p. 38), carcinoid syndrome (p. 234) etc.

C. CUTANEOUS MARKERS OF SYSTEMIC MALIGNANCY

There are many ways in which changes in the skin can indicate the possible presence of an underlying systemic malignancy.

1. Signs of exposure to a carcinogen

The significance of brown staining of the fingers due to cigarette smoking is unlikely to be missed in a patient with haemoptysis, but there are less well-known carcinogens which affect the skin.

Arsenic, widely used in the past for many skin, nerve and blood diseases, predisposes to internal malignancy, and it produces three distinct skin markers:

(i) Small circular brown keratoses of the palms and soles

(ii) Diffuse pigmentation with 'rain-drop' areas of paler normal skin.

(iii) Bowen's disease (p. 96) of the covered parts of the body.

X-irradiation of the spine, used in the past for ankylosing spondylitis, causes chronic radiation dermatitis and predisposes to leukaemia.

2. Direct involvement of the skin by malignant cells

Breast cancer commonly invades the skin directly and the 'peau d'orange' effect of lymph stasis is well-known. A rarer change is the erythematous plaque which resembles erysipelas (*carcinoma erysipeloides*).

Paget's disease of the nipple (p. 104) is well-known, but Paget's disease may also occur in the perineum as a sign of an underlying pelvic tumour.

Skin metastases are common in terminal cancer, but occasionally they are the presenting sign. Hypernephroma, which tends to be clinically occult, often metastasizes to the scalp as a solitary deposit, and treatment may give a prolonged remission.

Leukaemia and *malignant lymphoma* may also present with cutaneous infiltration (p. 103).

3. Miscellaneous signs of underlying malignancy

The commonest three skin markers of malignancy are *pallor*, due to anaemia, *pigmentation*, probably due to ectopic production of a melanocyte-stimulating hormone by the malignant cells, and generalized *pruritus*. The latter is particularly common with Hodgkin's disease, when it may be accompanied by eosinophilia.

Acanthosis nigricans is easily recognized as pigmented warty plaques with occur in the axillae and groins. It occasionally occurs as a familial disease starting in childhood, or as a complication of obesity or endocrine disease (especially acromegaly), but its development in a lean adult is sinister, since most of these patients have an adenocarcinoma of the gastro-intestinal tract. Occasionally the epidermal hyperplasia may also involve the neck and palms, and there may be papillomata of the gums.

Dermatomyositis (p. 221) in the adult indicates systemic malignancy in about 50 per cent of cases.

Herpes zoster is much less often due to malignancy, but nevertheless every patient should be fully examined, especially for evidence of a lymphoma. Other viral skin infection may also rarely become widespread due to the immune paresis of malignancy.

Clubbing (p. 53) may indicate bronchial carcinoma or mesothelioma. Occasionally this is accompanied by painful subperiosteal new bone formation (*hypertrophic pulmonary osteoarthropathy*) and rarely there is also marked thickening of the skin which is accompanied by seborrhoea and hyperhidrosis. The whole clinical picture is then called pachydermoperiostosis.

Many other associations between internal malignancy and the skin are known, but they are all rare:–

Erythema gyratum repens is a spectacular eruption in which figurate bands of erythema and scaling produce a widespread 'wood-grain' appearance. Recent work has shown this to be an immunological reaction to the underlying malignancy which is almost invariably present.

Another dramatic and reliable marker of malignancy is the sudden onset of fluffy blond hair growth over the whole face of an adult patient (*acquired hypertrichosis lanuginosa*).

The rapid onset of *multiple, irritable, seborrhoeic warts* has probably been over-emphasized in the past as a marker of malignancy, but despite the frequency of seborrhoeic warts in the ageing population, the possibility of malignancy must be carefully considered in such a case.

The sudden development of dry, scaly skin in middle life (*acquired ichthyosis*) is uncommon, and it often indicates an underlying lymphoma.

Carcinoma of the pancreas may occasionally present with cutaneous manifestations. Red, tender nodules of the legs may be due to *nodular panniculitis* secondary to circulating lipases, and these lesions can sometimes be difficult to distinguish from *superficial thrombophlebitis* which may also be due to pancreatic malignancy. If the neoplasm is in the head of the pancreas, *severe pruritus* may precede the other clinical signs of obstructive jaundice.

A *glucagonoma* is a rare malignant neoplasm of the pancreatic cells which produces a distinctive rash called *necrolytic migratory erythema* in response to the high levels of glucagon in the blood. These patients present with diabetes mellitus, glossitis, diarrhoea and blistering rash which usually spreads outwards from the perineum.

Another malignancy which produces a distinctive metabolic disturbance is the *carcinoid tumour* which causes *recurrent facial flushing*, often with permanent capillary dilatation, asthma and diarrhoea. Flushing can also be the presenting complaint of other forms of malignancy, and prostaglandins appear to be involved as the mediators of the flushing. In the carcinoid syndrome and in other malignancies, the flushing may be provoked by alcohol ingestion.

Leukaemia can involve the skin directly (p. 103) but it can also cause a rare distinctive rash which presents with scattered pustules, progressing to purple blistering lesions which become necrotic and ulcerate. This *bullous pyoderma gangrenosum* is not due to cutaneous infiltration by immature white cells, and it may even precede the circulating leucocytosis. A similar condition can occur in malignant myelomatosis.

Other bullous eruptions such as *pemphigus* (p. 199) and *pemphigoid* (p. 205) occur occasionally in patients with carcinoma, but epidemiological surveys have shown that the association is not significant. Isolated case-reports have, however, shown that a common antigen may be found in the skin and in the neoplasm, and occasionally the blisters clear following removal of the tumour. Presumably, therefore, carcinoma is one of the less frequent causes of auto-immune blistering disease.

4. Genetic syndromes predisposing to malignancy

Many inherited diseases are now known to predispose to the development of malignancy, and some of these have characteristic skin lesions which facilitate their recognition.

The *phakomatoses* are a group of diseases in which disseminated developmental defects affect the eyes, the skin and the nervous system. The best-known examples are *neurofibromatosis* (p. 112), associated with malignant glioma or phaeochromocytoma and *tuberous sclerosis* (p. 112), associated with rare neoplasia such as the rhabdomyosarcoma.

Familial polyposis coli (Gardner's syndrome) is another dominant disease. The multiple polyps in the colon have a high incidence of malignant degeneration and prophylactic colonectomy may be advisable in affected subjects. Some but not all patients have multiple epidermoid cysts (wens) on the face and scalp, with bone cysts in the jaw, and these two features in a hitherto undiagnosed patient should suggest the need for colonoscopy.

Peutz-Jegher's syndrome is the association of peri-oral lentiginosis (small brown spots around the mouth) with multiple small intestinal polyps. These commonly cause intussusception during the teens, but they virtually never become malignant. A few patients however also have polyps in the stomach or colon and these may become carcinomatous in later life.

Defective immunosurveillance refers to a defect in immune competence which allows malignant cells to evade detection and destruction by the immune system. Several rare inherited diseases with defects in immunological competence have an increased risk of malignancy, and some of these produce cutaneous markers. The best known example is the *Wiskott-Aldrich syndrome* with eczema, and purpura due to thrombocytopenia.

SYSTEMIC EFFECTS OF CUTANEOUS DISEASE

The preceding sections of this chapter have indicated the wide variety of cutaneous changes that may be produced by systemic disease, but it must also be remembered that internal organs may conversely be affected by widespread skin desease, and in erythroderma these systemic effects of skin disease may assume major importance.

Erythroderma ('exfoliative dermatitis')

This term is applied to any inflammatory skin disease which affects more than 90 per cent of the body surface. In these cases there is usually a uniform scaly erythema and until the disease is controlled it is often impossible to be sure of the underlying cause. There is often a widespread pitting oedema, and facial oedema often causes eversion of the eye-lids (ectropion), with resulting conjunctivitis. There may be severe hair loss. The commonest causes of erythroderma are *eczema, psoriasis, drug allergy* and *lymphoma or leukemia*.

Systemic effects of erythroderma.

Before steroids were available, erythroderma was fatal in about one third of cases, and heart failure and pneumonia were commonly listed as the cause of death. Fatalities in non-malignant cases are now rare but attention must be paid to the following factors:

1. *Haemodynamic effects.* In erythroderma the cutaneous capillary bed is fully dilated and the skin feels hot due to the increased blood flow. There is often tachycardia and a collapsing pulse, and the cardiac output is sometimes increased. Much of the cardiac output is diverted to the skin, and the blood-flow to other organs may be diminished. The plasma volume is increased, and there is often widespread cutaneous oedema due to increased capillary permeability and hypoalbuminaemia.

2. *Thermoregulation.* Erythrodermic patients often behave almost like 'cold-blooded' animals and show alarming fluctuations in temperature according to their environment. In a cold room they may become hypothermic, since they are unable to vasoconstrict their skin vessels. A low-reading thermometer must be used to detect this, since of course the skin does not feel cold to the touch. Patients kept under blankets in a warm room will become hyperpyrexial, because the basal metabolic rate is increased. The inflamed skin may produce a circulating pyrogen, and the hypothalamic 'thermostat' becomes abnormal, so that inappropriate shivering occurs.

3. *Haematological effects.* These include anaemia, leucocytosis and raised ESR. Folate deficiency is common (usually due to malabsorption) and the serum iron is decreased, but this is usually a metabolic effect, not a true deficiency of iron. Protein metabolism is also abnormal. Plasma albumin is decreased due to hypervolaemia, increased capillary permeability and increased protein loss through the bowel and skin (desquamation). Plasma globulins are often increased, but the cause of this is obscure.

4. *Fluid balance.* Both thirst and oliguria are common in erythroderma. This positive fluid balance presumably compensates for the increased transepidermal water loss and the plasma loss from increased capillary permeability.

5. *Intestinal effects* Erythroderma is sometimes associated with malabsorption and this abnormality is reversed by successful treatment of the inflamed skin. There may also be a protein-losing enteropathy. This 'dermatogenic enteropathy' must be distinguished from the coeliac disease associated with dermatitis herpetiformis, which is not secondary to the rash.

6. *Lymphadenopathy* The lymph nodes in the axillae and groins are usually considerably enlarged in erythroderma of any cause, and many cases have in the past been misdiagnosed as lymphoma. On

biopsy however their normal architecture is preserved, and they contain quantities of melanin and fat derived from the inflamed skin.

7. *Miscellaneous metabolic effects*

(i) Gynaecomastia is a common finding in chronic erythroderma and some patients have increased urinary oestrogens.

(ii) Hyperuricaemia is a feature of erythrodermic psoriasis due to the increased cell turnover.

(iii) Hypocalcaemia is probably secondary to the decreased plasma albumin or to malabsorption.

Treatment of erythroderma

Topical steroids form the mainstay of treatment, but in life-threatening cases systemic steroids may also be used.

21

The skin and the psyche

The role of psychological factors in causing or aggravating skin disease is controversial. Much nonsense has been written on this subject in the past, and this uncritical and uncontrolled work has produced a reaction among some dermatologists against psychosomatic concepts which may not be entirely justified.

It has been claimed by some psychoanalysts, for example, that pruritus vulvae is due to repressed nymphomania, and pruritus ani is a sign of latent homosexuality. The fact that pruritus vulvae often disappears when the Candida is treated, and pruritus ani may vanish with the thread worms does not appear to diminish the religious fervour of their beliefs. The treatment of the Id by the odd? At the other extreme are those scientific purists who believe that skin diseases are due entirely to biochemical factors, and if a phenomenon cannot be scientifically demonstrated then it probably does not exist. The views of most dermatologists lie somewhere between these extremes. They are impressed by the fact that psychological 'tension' (whatever that is) appears to have an adverse effect on some skin diseases such as eczema and acne even though it cannot yet be measured.

Strictly speaking, a psychosomatic disease should fulfil two criteria:

1. It should be predictably reproduced by psychic stimulation.
2. It should be healed or prevented by psychotherapy.

It is doubtful whether any skin diseases other than excessive blushing and sweating fulfil these criteria. The psychotherapy of skin disease, even when performed by a trained psychiatrist for a 'psychosomatic' disorder such as dermatitis artefacta, seems to give singularly poor results, and the best-controlled study to date on the role of the psychiatrist in the treatment of eczema showed that psychiatric intervention actually had an adverse effect on the skin disease.

The following diseases however are generally accepted to be psychological in origin:

1. Dermatitis artefacta

This term refers to skin lesions which are self-inflicted, with no obvious underlying cause such as pruritus (Fig. 21.1). A wide variety of physical and chemical methods of damaging the skin may be used, and patients can be very cunning in disguising their activities. One classical presentation is self-inflicted lymphoedema due to intermittent application of a tourniquet. Occasionally there is an obvious material gain to the patient, e.g., infliction of 'sores' by vagabonds to gain admission to hospital, or prevention of wound healing to increase an insurance claim, but more often there is no apparent cause, and patients will strenuously deny producing the

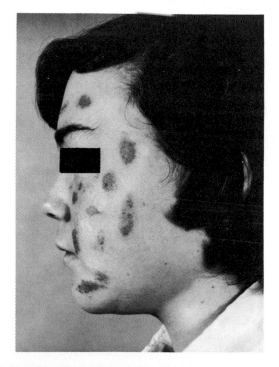

Fig. 21.1 Dermatitis artefacta. These lesions developed simultaneously over a period of 2 hours

lesions even when 'caught in the act'. The diagnosis is usually suggested by the bizarre shape of the lesions, their sudden appearance, and their failure to respond to therapy except under occlusive dressings and constant supervision. The patients are characteristically complacent about lesions which may look most alarming to the observer ('la belle indifference', also known as the Mona Lisa smile).

Dermatitis artefacta is a dangerous diagnosis to make, for once the label is attached, the patient loses credibility and several diseases such as porphyria cutanea tarda and vasculitis can simulate artefacts. Most patients with dermatitis artefacta are insecure young women. They tend to be mentally or sexually immature, often with a dominant or aggressive mother. Sometimes the skin problems represent only a part of a clinical spectrum along with simulated pyrexia, hysterical aphonia, drug overdose etc., which represent a non-verbal 'cry for help'. The response to any kind of treatment (even from a psychiatrist) is usually poor. The essence of management is to maintain sympathetic contact with the patient, but not to alienate her by confrontation with the diagnosis. One can, however, hint that the skin lesions must be due to some external agency, and the patients seem to understand this subtle relationship.

Religious 'stigmata' can also be classed as a self-inflicted skin disease. The lesions appear as spontaneous purpura or bleeding on the forehead, linear weals or ecchymoses on the back, and bloody tears or sweat. Those afflicted are usually devout Catholics with a hysterical personality, and the lesions appear following a period of fasting or religious fervour, especially in Holy Week.

'Spontaneous bruising' also occurs occasionally in the irreligious. Skin tests have shown evidence of 'erythrocyte auto-sensitization' in some patients, but many dermatologists believe the lesions are often self-inflicted.

Tattoos

These are a special form of self-inflicted skin lesion, and several studies have shown that they tend to be associated with personality disorders, or criminal behaviour. As a tattooist once remarked 'Yeah doc, business is fine, but nothing to what it would be if I could remove them'. Tattoos can be removed by skin grafting or by salabrasion, in which table salt is scrubbed into the anaesthetized skin, and the hypertonic irritant solution disperses the pigment particles. This can produce scars however, and there is no guarantee that the patient will not have further tattoos performed.

2. Cutaneous hypochondriasis ('dermatological non-disease')

In this condition there is an obsession with a trivial skin blemish such as 'dilated pores' or clinically inapparent 'baldness'. Sometimes this is evidence of a psychosis such as schizophrenia, but more often, especially in middle-aged women, it probably reflects a feeling of insecurity, due for example to marital discord.

These patients often require an inordinately long consultation and they tend to become angry if reassurance is offered. Many of them are depressed, and may even become suicidal, but they generally reject the idea of psychiatric referral because they are convinced that it is their skin (or hair, or nose, or breast size) which is their only problem. Some of these patients will respond to treatment with prolonged psychotherapy (preferably from a handsome young doctor with a slightly foreign accent) or to a combination of treatment with pimozide and antidepressant. Many drift into the murkier realms of private practice and others cure themselves by starting an affair with the milkman.

3. Delusions of infestation ('parasitophobia')

These interesting folk believe for no good reason that their skin is infested with parasites or insects. They will often complain of a sensation of itching, crawling or 'gnawing' of the skin, and they often gouge out small pieces of skin which they keep safely wrapped up or bottled until the next clinic visit, when the desiccated debris is triumphantly produced for the doctor to identify. The delusion is often so strong that other people may become convinced of the danger of infestation, and they may take great precautions to prevent this. Neighbouring scientists, veterinary surgeons or museum curators may be involved in fruitless attempts to catch and identify the parasite. The record stands at 'folie à quatre' in a psychiatrist's family. Many patients with this delusion are obviously psychotic and it is important that organic causes of psychosis (B_{12} deficiency, frontal lobe tumour, etc.) are excluded. The doctor must also recall that an odd personality does not prevent a patient developing a genuine infestation. Patients with 'parasitophobia' often respond dramatically to treatment with the psychotropic drug pimozide.

As stated earlier, many other diseases are believed by many experienced dermatologists to be exacerbated or occasionally precipitated by psychological factors, even though they may have a biochemical explanation at a cellular level. The list of such diseases varies with the individual, but usually includes:

1. Most forms of pruritus (including atopic eczema, seborrhoeic dermatitis and lichen simplex)
2. Urticaria
3. Hyperhidrosis
4. Lichen planus
5. Alopecia areata
6. Vitiligo
7. Herpes simplex

The effect of stress and other emotional factors on the skin has been little studied. The acute effects mediated by emotionally-induced vascular and neurological changes are a matter of common observation ('white with rage', 'red with shame', 'cold sweat of fear', 'goose-pimples' etc.) but the more subtle effects of stress on the immune system etc. are poorly understood. It may be significant that experiments in the NASA Skylab programme have demonstrated depressed lymphocyte transformation on the day of splashdown, presumably due to the effect of stress, and depressed lymphocyte function has also been demonstrated following bereavement.

Even if the effect of the psyche on skin disease is controversial there is no doubt that skin disease often has a profound effect on the psyche. Many patients become depressed and worried by their disease, and the degree of psychological upset often bears no relation to the objective severity of their disease. Every medical consultation should involve some degree of psychotherapy, and most patients will benefit from reassurance and explanation. Patients often have a feeling of guilt or a fear of cancer or contagious disease which can easily be removed, but in some cases, especially where there is objective cause for worry and depression (e.g., loss of a job due to severe eczema) it may be necessary to use tranquillizers or anti-depressants.

22

Drug reactions

A typical 'drug eruption' is easy to recognise. It is a widespread symmetrical, blotchy, urticated or morbilliform rash usually affecting the trunk. It is of sudden onset, and is often accompanied by a pyrexia. It is important to realize however that many cases are atypical, and many other morphological appearances can occur (pustules, blisters, purpura, pigmentation, etc.). Drug-induced disease has become more common with increasing medication of the population, and drug reactions have now replaced syphilis as the great mimic of other diseases.

The history is vital, and every doctor who refers a patient for diagnosis should record in his referral letter *all* the drugs which the patient has recently received. Allergy to a drug can suddenly develop after several years of trouble-free medication, and there is probably no drug which *never* causes a reaction. Even intelligent patients are often surprisingly vague about their drug history, and will forget that they take purgatives, or analgesics for headaches, period pains, etc. even when specifically questioned. The questions must be repeated, and it is amazing how often patients will cheerfully admit to the consultant what they had strenuously denied to the house-officer a few hours earlier

Unfortunately there is still no reliable skin test for a drug reaction. Prick tests and patch tests are sometimes used, but there are many false positives and false negatives. If the rash has been mild it is sometimes possible to confirm the diagnosis by giving a 'challenge' dose of the drug at a later date. There is the danger however that subsequent reactions may be much more severe, particularly with Type 1 ('immediate') reactions. It is vitally important that drugs such as penicillin should not be administered by injection to a patient who gives a history of previous urticaria due to the drug, as there is a risk that a fatal 'anaphylactic shock' may be produced. A drug rash should normally clear within a week or two of stopping the drug, but a gold eruption can persist for six months or more after the last injection.

It is important that a drug should be stopped if it is seriously suspected to be causing a hypersensitivity reaction, since if it is continued it may cause renal or hepatic damage.

Clinical patterns

The following incomplete list gives some idea of the diversity of cutaneous drug reactions:

1. *Urticated or morbilliform rash* Antibiotics, etc.
2. *Erythroderma* Barbiturates, etc.
3. *Blisters* Barbiturate overdose, etc. (Fig. 22.1)
4. *Stevens-Johnson syndrome and toxic epidermal necrolysis* Long-acting sulphonamides, etc.
5. *Purpura and ecchymoses* (i) Carbromal, etc.
   (ii) Drugs causing thrombocytopenia
6. *Erythema nodosum* Sulphonamides

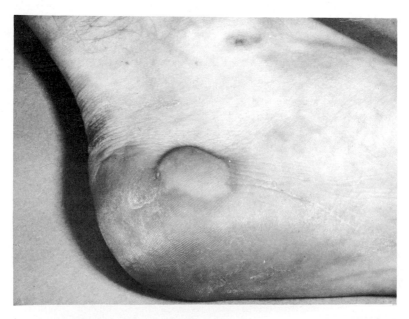

Fig. 22.1 A blister on a pressure point following barbiturate-induced coma

7. *Photosensitivity* Phenothiazines, etc. (p. 160)
8. *Lichen Planus* Antimalarials, etc.
9. *Acne vulgaris* Androgens, etc.
10. *Acneiform pustules* Iodides, glucocorticoids etc. (Fig. 22.2).
11. *Livedo reticulosis* Amantadine
12. *Pigmentation* Busulphan, amiodarone etc.
13. *Hypertrichosis* Diazoxide, minoxidil
14. *Hirsutism* Androgens, anabolic steroids
15. *Alopecia* Cytotoxic drugs, etc.
16. *Lupus erythematosus* Procainamide, etc.
17. *Psoriasiform* Practolol
18. *'Fixed drug eruption'* This is a special pattern of drug rash in which the inflammation is localized to the same area of skin every time the drug is taken. Between attacks the affected skin is characteristically pigmented. Phenolphthalein is a well-known cause, and the relationship between a recurrent patch of inflamed skin and laxative ingestion is often missed.

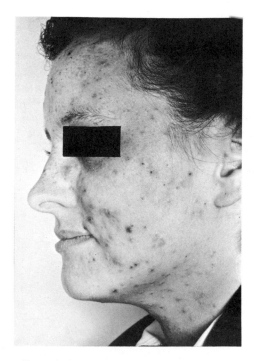

Fig. 22.2 An acneiform drug rash

Mechanisms of drug reactions

Most drug rashes are presumed to be due to the development of hypersensitivity. Any type of allergic reaction can occur, but the immunological mechanism in individual cases is usually obscure.

Sometimes the reaction is pharmacological rather than immunological, and it may be either a predictable side-effect (e.g., alopecia with large doses of cytotoxics) or an idiosyncratic reaction (e.g., urticaria with aspirin).

The ampicillin rash is of particular interest. Patients who present with a sore throat due to infectious mononucleosis are sometimes treated (wrongly) with ampicillin and over 90 per cent of such patients develop a typical drug rash. If the ampicillin is given following recovery from the infectious mononucleosis it no longer causes a rash, presumably because the patient's immune status has changed.

Cross-sensitization

If a subject is sensitized to a drug, a reaction may sometimes be produced by a different but chemically related compound. This may be an obvious relationship e.g., between different penicillins, or it may be more subtle e.g., sulphonamides and some local anaesthetics which share the para-amino group. Sometimes the original sensitization may have been due to a topical application, and subsequent ingestion of a related chemical may then produce a severe reaction with erythroderma. Hair dyes and sulphonamides cross-react in this way.

23

Principles of treatment

Many people have an instinctive loathing of skin diseases, and the success of the modern cosmetics industry testifies to the fact that even minor cutaneous blemishes are not gladly tolerated. Because skin disease is visible, and patients are so demanding, there is a great temptation to be over-zealous in treatment. Common examples of overtreatment include the application of irritants, sensitizers (especially antihistamine or local anaesthetic creams) or potent steroids for trivial self-limiting conditions. It is also tempting to use potentially toxic systemic therapy (steroids, immunosuppressives, hormones, etc.) for conditions which, though unremitting, may be no more than a cosmetic defect. At the other extreme, some doctors seem to consider all skin diseases as too trivial to be worth treating. A curt dismissal is just as bad as overtreatment, for even a mild cosmetic defect can sometimes cause considerable psychological anguish or even suicide. A careful weighing of the pros and cons of each treatment is always required, taking the patient's personality, occupation and social background into account. Holistic medicine is nowhere more important than in dermatology.

Most skin diseases can be successfully treated by a relatively small number of simple preparations, and it is better to become experienced in the use of a few preparations, rather than to be always trying the latest nostrum, even if you do need a new ball-point pen. In many cases, *how* a preparation is used is just as important as *what* is used, and careful explanation to the patient is always worthwhile (people can do the most extraordinary things with nystatin pessaries). The doctor must also be aware that self-treatment is common, and neighbours will pass tubes of 'Wondercream' over the fence if the ointment left over from Granny's shingles has not worked. The patient should always be asked what he or she has been putting on the skin, and one should also, of course, ask about other medication, including purgatives, headache powders, analgesics for 'period pains' etc.

Environmental factors are also important, and advice must be given in appropriate cases about avoidance of heat, cold, allergens, over-frequent bathing, poor hygiene, detergents, woollen clothing, etc.

LOCAL THERAPY

As a result of exhortations about over prescribing, doctors commonly underestimate the amount of medicament required to treat a skin disease, and patients frequently complain that 'the rash came back when the ointment ran out'. A single application of ointment to the entire body surface of an adult requires 30 g, and a similar application of a lotion applied on gauze requires about 150 ml.

Bases

Drugs applied to the skin are usually dissolved or suspended in a base (vehicle). The choice of base is extremely important, because it not only governs the degree of penetration of the drug into the skin and its clearance into the systemic circulation, but it also has a vital influence regarding the risk of side-effects (sensitization, stinging, etc.), the degree of protection provided against adverse environmental effects (irritant chemicals, etc.) and its cosmetic acceptability (greasiness, smell, etc.). In addition, ointment bases (e.g. lanolin) and preservatives (e.g. parabens) can cause allergic reactions and so prevent an eczema from responding to treatment.

Penetration

Drugs may penetrate the skin by three routes: (1) They can cross the epidermal cells directly, by penetrating the cell membranes to enter and leave the cytoplasm. (2) They can penetrate the interstices between the cells without crossing the cell membrane. (3) They can use the channels provided by the sweat ducts and the hair follicles.
  The physico-chemical considerations which determine the relative importance of each route at different levels in the skin are obviously extremely complex but, in practice, it is the stratum corneum of the epidermis which offers the major barrier to penetration.
  The chosen formulation should aim to deliver the drug at the 'right' level in the skin, as the following examples illustrate:

1 *Skin surface* (no penetration) e.g. sunscreens, insect repellants.

2. *Stratum corneum* e.g., anti-fungal preparations.
3. *Epidermis and dermis* e.g., topical steroids for eczema.
4. *Sebaceous glands* e.g., topical antibiotics for acne.
5. *Sweat glands* e.g., antiperspirants.
6. *Systemic absorption* e.g., glyceryl trinitrate for angina.

Most drug firms spend considerable sums of money assessing the absorption kinetics and distribution of their topical preparations. This can be achieved by a variety of techniques, such as the assay of a biological endpoint (e.g., vasoconstrictor assay for steroids), the measured disappearance of the drug from the skin surface, serial analysis of the appearance of the drug in the blood or urine, and autoradiography of the radio-labelled drug in a skin biopsy.

Composition of bases

Bases contain one or more of the following constituents mixed in various proportions: water, alcohol, grease, and powder. Bases used alone may have a beneficial effect in some skin conditions:

(i) *Powders* Dusting powders can be used in skin folds to lessen friction and to repel or to absorb moisture, (e.g., starch powder, zinc oxide powder, talcum powder)

(ii) *Watery lotions* These cool inflamed areas by evaporation. The cooling effect may be hastened by adding an alcohol, or retarded by the addition of glycerol or arachis oil. Substances which precipitate protein (astringents) may be added to decrease exudates

(iii) *Shake lotions* These are watery lotions to which powder has been added to increase the area available for evaporation. Their disadvantage is that during drying the powder may clump together to form abrasive particles.

(iv) *Creams* These are emulsions of water and grease which are used for their moisturizing and emollient effects. Generally an oil-in-water emulsion (e.g., aqueous cream BPC) is better absorbed and therefore feels less greasy than a water-in-oil emulsion (e.g., oil cream BPC). The former are sometimes called 'vanishing creams', and the latter are 'cooling creams'. The emulsifying agents (e.g. wool alcohols) and preservatives (e.g. parabens) which must be added to creams may sensitize some patients and cause eczema.

Ointments

These are greasy preparations which are occlusive and emollient, so that they are particularly useful for dry, scaly conditions which are made worse by external irritants, e.g. industrial dermatitis. They retain moisture in the skin by preventing evaporation of water from the stratum corneum (trans-epidermal water loss).

Pastes

These are usually powders mixed with a grease or oil. They are protective and emollient, and a pink paste (e.g., zinc compound paste BPC) can be used to disguise an unsightly rash, but they tend to be messy unless covered by a dressing.

Topical steroids

These deserve special mention because of their widespread use and potential dangers. There is no doubt that steroid ointments have improved the quality of life for millions of patients. Like most other potent drugs however, they have several side-effects and several fatalities and numerous cosmetic disasters have occurred due to their injudicious use. Such patients have sometimes been given numerous repeat prescriptions for a potent steroid ointment without adequate supervision and with no warning of the dangers of prolonged usage. Potent topical steroids should be used with the same care as oral prednisone.

What is a potent topical steroid?

It is difficult to rank glucocorticoids in exact order of potency since the results vary according to which particular biological test is used e.g., the vasoconstrictor test result does not always coincide with clinical efficacy, which in any case may vary with the disease being treated. For practical purposes however clinical potency correlates closely with the potential for harmful side-effects, irrespective of whether the molecule is fluorinated or not.

The following preparations are regarded as *very potent*:
Beclomethasone dipropionate 0.5% ('Propaderm Forte')
Clobetasol propionate 0.05% ('Dermovate')
Fluocinolone acetonide 0.20% ('Synalar Forte')
Diflucortolone valerate 0.3% ('Nerisone Forte')
Halcinonide 0.1% ('Halciderm')

The following preparations are mild, and are regarded as being unlikely to produce serious side-effects:
Hydrocortisone base or acetate 0.1% to 2%

Clobetasone butyrate 0.05% ('Eumovate')
Flurandrenolone 0.0125% ('Haelan')
Fluocinolone acetonide 0.01% ('Synandone')
Methylprednisolone 0.25% ('Medrone').

Most other preparations ('Betnovate', 'Diprosone', 'Propaderm', 'Synalar', etc.) would be placed somewhere between these extremes.

Side-effects of potent topical glucocorticoids

1. Cutaneous atrophy

The loss of dermal collagen, which is dose-related, causes the skin to become thin and fragile. The lack of connective tissue support causes capillary dilatation and easy bruising. Unsightly purple striae may develop, particularly in areas under tension, such as the back and thighs. Potent steroids applied regularly to the face will produce a plethoric complexion (Fig. 23.1), and they may precipitate peri-oral dermatitis. They will make rosacea worse in the long term

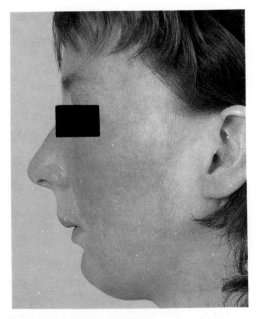

Fig. 23.1 Facial erythema due to prolonged use of a potent topical steroid

(p. 66), and if applied to venous ulcers they will enlarge them (Fig. 23.2).

2. Infection

Bacterial infection is more likely in steroid-treated skin, particularly if the area is rendered warm and moist by occlusion. Care is also needed when treating the body folds (e.g. groins and sub-mammary areas) as these regions are also warm and moist.

The spread of fungal infections is also facilitated by topical steroids, and their diagnosis is hampered because of the altered appearance of the rash (Fig. 23.3).

3. Systemic effects

Application of potent steroids to large areas of skin can produce enough systemic absorption to suppress the adrenal glands. The absorption is enhanced by cutaneous inflammation, and by the use

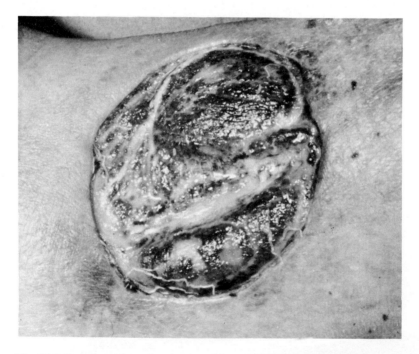

Fig. 23.2 Leg ulcer 'cleaned' and enlarged by application of a potent steroid ointment

of polythene occlusion. Steroids are degraded in the liver, and in patients with hepatic dysfunction steroid ointments may cause the same side-effects as systemic prednisone. Infants are also at particular risk from systemic absorption.

The prolonged use of potent topical steroids is therefore inadvisable in the following conditions:

1. Infancy
2. Most facial dermatoses
3. Widespread inflammatory skin disease
4. Hepatic failure
5. Infected dermatoses, unless 'covered' by the simultaneous use of the appropriate antibiotic.

If a rash can be controlled only by the prolonged use of potent steroids, the diagnosis should be reviewed to make sure that conditions such as photosensitivity, drug reaction and contact dermatitis

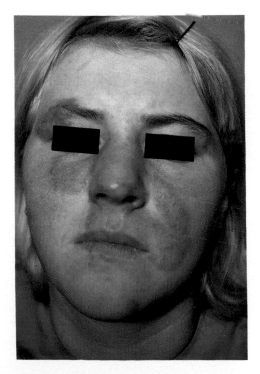

Fig. 23.3 Tinea incognita. The atypical appearance of a dermatophyte treated by a topical steroid

are not being missed. Occasionally the acarus isolated in the dermatology clinic has a moon-face and a buffalo hump!

Combination therapy

Topical steroids are often combined with one or more preparations such as antiseptics or antibiotics. There is certainly a place for combination therapy in conditions such as infected eczema, or seborrhoeic dermatitis of the flexures, but the novice should resist the temptation always to use 'blunderbuss' therapy in order to obviate the need for accurate diagnosis. A general practitioner of my acquaintance classified skin diseases into three types: (1) those that itch, (2) those that look ugly, (3) those that smell. This classification was too complex for therapeutic purposes though, and was revised to two types: (1) those that respond to 'Dermovate NN' (a combination of a very potent steroid with neomycin and nystatin), (2) those that do not. This approach is not to be encouraged.

Index